BIOTECHNOLOGY IN AGRICULTURE, INDUSTRY AND MEDICINE

IN VIVO IMAGING

NEW RESEARCH

BIOTECHNOLOGY IN AGRICULTURE, INDUSTRY AND MEDICINE

Additional books in this series can be found on Nova's website under the Series tab.

Additional e-books in this series can be found on Nova's website under the e-book tab.

BIOTECHNOLOGY IN AGRICULTURE, INDUSTRY AND MEDICINE

IN VIVO IMAGING

NEW RESEARCH

RICK HOUGH
AND
JARED CAMARILLO
EDITORS

New York

For permission to use material from this book please contact us:
Telephone 631-231-7269; Fax 631-231-8175
Web Site: http://www.novapublishers.com

NOTICE TO THE READER

Additional color graphics may be available in the e-book version of this book.

Library of Congress Cataloging-in-Publication Data

ISBN: 978-1-62948-633-8

Library of Congress Control Number: 2013955181

Published by Nova Science Publishers, Inc. † New York

Contents

Preface

In this book, the authors present current research in the study of in vivo imaging. Topics discussed include nuclear magnetic resonance imaging of metabolites in plants and animals; the design and application of magnetic-based theranostic nanoparticle systems, an investigation on their potentially harmful effects and an exploration of their future role in personalized medicine; an overview of techniques for in vivo bone imaging, including X-ray, micro-computed tomography, magnetic resonance imaging; SPECT/PET nuclear imaging technologies, and ultrasound; and the in vivo imaging of the central nervous system anatomy, fiber connectivity and functional activity.

Chapter 1 – This review highlights technological developments in magnetic resonance imaging (MRI), which are creating opportunities for the visualization and quantification of metabolites in plant and animal materials. Some of the leading MRI-based strategies for metabolite imaging are explained, and peculiarities of MRI application on plant and animal (as experimental models) are highlighted. A major feature of MRI is that it is a non-invasive platform, and thus can be used for the analysis of living organisms. By concentrating on plants, the authors explore the opportunities offered, and the challenges posed by MRI for elucidating the metabolism of living organisms. Here, the aim is to convince the reader of the need to develop non-invasive approaches to study plant metabolism, and in particular to demonstrate the merits of MRI for this purpose. The authors suggest that a co-operative effort between MRI physicists and plant biologists will yield a substantial research significant dividend.

Chapter 2 – The publicity of recently introduced nanoparticles is accelerating in the constantly developing field of cancer research; nanotechnology is being increasingly utilized for the development of breakthrough approaches in terms of cancer diagnosis and therapy. Magnetic nanoparticles offer unprecedented prospect for magnetic separation, nanoparticle-enhanced hyperthermia, targeted drug delivery, regenerative medicine and stem cell therapy and as contrast agents. Magnetic resonance imaging (MRI) is an important medical imaging tool, which has the ability to incorporate such contrast agents and provide enhanced clinical information with high spatial and temporal resolutions. Due to its nonionizing radiation, high sensitivity to the distribution of water and other biomolecules and the orientation of fine tissue structures, MRI has been widely applied in clinical practice. Given the recent progress in nanosynthesis and bioengineering, magnetic nanoparticles are expected to serve as an innovative platform, which will enable novel approaches to targeted tumor imaging and therapy. Not only the fabrication of nanoparticles that combine multimodality methods will discard many inadequacies that are present in single-modality imaging methods but also the incorporation of cancer-specific therapeutic payloads will equip these nanoparticles with the ability to provide magnetic-field dependent drug delivery. It is however imperative that, prior to the application of mangetic-based theranostic nanoparticle systems in clinical settings, several key issues need to be addressed, including toxicity, long-term stability and distribution. The aim of this review is to present the latest developments in the design and application of mangetic-based theranostic nanoparticle systems, investigate on their potentially harmful events and explore their future role in personalized medicine.

Chapter 3 – Bone is a specialised connective tissue comprising of cells and bone matrix. The two main constituents of bone are an inorganic mineralised component and a highly organised collagen organic component. It responds to stimuli such as mechanical forces, hormone levels and disease. Unlike the other connective tissues, the extracellular matrix of bone is mineralised, making it a hard, unyielding substance ideally suited for its supportive and protective functions. Depending on the location, different types of bone are different in structure and shape, which can be apparent when bone is imaged.

Non-invasive *in vivo* imaging of bone can be a useful tool for the diagnosis and assessment of bone quality, allowing the monitoring of the bone in real time during physiological/pathological events such as fractures, disease, healing and remodelling. Discovered over 100 years ago, the most commonly used method for bone imaging is still X-ray spectroscopy. Since then, many new techniques have been developed. For *in vivo* work, this will increase the quality of the outcome (via self-comparative studies) and reduce the number of animals required, with advantageous economic and ethical implications.

This chapter provides an overview of techniques for *in vivo* bone imaging, including the better established methods of X-ray, micro computed tomography, magnetic resonance imaging, SPECT/PET nuclear imaging technologies and ultrasound. It also covers some more modern and less prevalent methods, such as fluorescence and bioluminescent. The advantages, limitations and indications of the application of each technique are also discussed.

Chapter 4 – Imaging distinct neuronal networks and testing their functionality *in vivo* is challenging. While conventional magnetic resonance imaging (MRI) that is based on tissue-specific water relaxation provides detailed insight into the structural organization of the brain, manganese-enhanced MRI (MEMRI) affords additional layers of information regarding cellular composition, functional connectivity and activity within the CNS. Pioneered by A.P. Koretsky in 1998, it has emerged as a highly versatile and reliable tool for qualitative and quantitative neuroimaging. The expansion of MEMRI applications has been promoted by the increase in transgenic mouse models and the sophisticated technical progress achieved for small rodent MRI. The technique exploits the paramagnetic properties of manganese (Mn^{2+}), which augments MR contrast mainly by shortening the T_1 spin-lattice relaxation time. As a calcium (Ca^{2+}) analog, it is incorporated into neurons by voltage-gated Ca^{2+} channels and actively transported along the axonal cytoskeleton. While Mn^{2+} accumulates in synaptic target areas, trans-synaptic propagation and re-uptake into secondary or tertiary neuronal circuits are limited. Thus, MEMRI represents a highly selective *in vivo* method for imaging brain anatomy, fiber connectivity, and neuronal activity with low unintentional background signaling. Mn^{2+} can be delivered by systemic administration for imaging neuroarchitectural features and mapping active brain areas or applied topically, e.g. via intranasal and intraocular microinjections to visualize primary sensory projections. In such studies, Mn^{2+}-dependent signal enhancement within axonal target regions represents a quantitative measure for structural integrity and metabolic viability of axonal connection, e.g. during post-traumatic de- and reorganization of axonal fibers and for assessing axonal transport impairments after genetic or pharmacological interventions. For each application, MEMRI protocols detailing optimized dose-responses for individual animal models are available, thus enabling repetitive and longitudinal *in vivo* studies without Mn^{2+} toxicity. Given the broad spectrum of MEMRI applications, this chapter serves as a useful and informative introduction for new users, but also will be of interest to more experienced operators. The chapter further discusses currently unresolved questions and future perspectives of MEMRI. For example, the observation that signal enhancement along the retino-tectal projection is unaffected in poor-sighted mice raises important questions about the electrophysiological properties that affect neuronal uptake and axonal transport of Mn^{2+}. Exciting technical modifications are presently underway that will further promote the applicability of MEMRI. One approach is working towards the precipitation of Mn^{2+} by autometallography to combine *in toto* MRI of CNS structures with the histological detection of Mn^{2+} at the cellular level. Other MEMRI studies have already demonstrated that Mn^{2+} toxicity can be reduced by topical delivery as eye drops or by safe circulatory release from Mn^{2+} derivatives. Thus, diagnostic applications to monitor cerebral functions and neuropathological alterations in humans are envisaged in the near future.

In: *In Vivo* Imaging: New Research
Editors: R. Hough and J. Camarillo
ISBN: 978-1-62948-633-8

Chapter 1

Nuclear Magnetic Resonance Imaging of Metabolites in Plants and Animals

Ljudmilla Borisjuk[1]* and Gerd Melkus[2]
[1]Leibniz-Institute of Plant Genetics and Crop Plant Research (IPK), Gatersleben, Germany
[2]Dept. of Medical Imaging, The Ottawa Hospital, Civic Campus, Ottawa, ON, Canada

Abstract

This review highlights technological developments in magnetic resonance imaging (MRI), which are creating opportunities for the visualization and quantification of metabolites in plant and animal materials. Some of the leading MRI-based strategies for metabolite imaging are explained, and peculiarities of MRI application on plant and animal (as experimental models) are highlighted. A major feature of MRI is that it is a non-invasive platform, and thus can be used for the analysis of living organisms. By concentrating on plants, we explore the opportunities offered, and the challenges posed by MRI for elucidating the metabolism of living organisms. Here, the aim is to convince the reader of the need to develop non-invasive approaches to study plant

* E-mail address: borysyuk@ipk-gatersleben.de.

metabolism, and in particular to demonstrate the merits of MRI for this purpose. We suggest that a co-operative effort between MRI physicists and plant biologists will yield a substantial research significant dividend.

Introduction

Making sense of visual signals directly or indirectly occupies about 50% of the brain's processing power, and the brain is able to processes information from images more effectively than from other sources (Smiciklas, 2012). The capacity of NMR (Nuclear Magnetic Resonance) to generate images, which commonly regarded to the term "Magnetic Resonance Imaging" (MRI), was discovered over 40 years ago and since this time the platform has evolved into a powerful method for imaging live biological material. The specific properties which suit it so well as a tool for the *in vivo* study of metabolites are highlighted in this review.

MRI is non-invasive technique, meaning that the images can be generated without any need to process the target tissue. Doing away with sample extraction and/or purification avoids many of the artefacts associated with conventional analytical methods. Secondly, the platform permits the detection of some processes which are not assayable *in vitro*, as for example, real time variation in the structure and chemistry of the living cell. Thirdly, the platform generates multi-faceted (simultaneously spectroscopic, spatial and dynamic) data, a property which is particularly valuable in the context of live specimens, since it allows for a wide-ranging monitoring of function from a single experiment. (In contrast, most conventional analytical methods require the investigator to focus on a narrow set of parameters, such as either "structure" or "metabolism"). The combination of these advantages has helped to turn MRI into a highly versatile medical diagnostics platform technology, but its implementation in the plant sciences is not as yet so advanced.

The early NMR-acquired images of both human (Hinshaw et al., 1977; Mansfield and Maudsley, 1977) and plant (Hinshaw et al., 1979; Mansfeld and Pykett, 1978) materials were published approximately simultaneously, but the impact within the two scientific communities has been rather different. Following the early suggestion that NMR could be adopted as a platform for cancer diagnosis (Damadian, 1971), large numbers of MRI systems were installed in hospitals throughout the world. A clinical device provided the means for the earliest documented applications of MRI in the plant sciences (Mansfield and Pykett, 1978; Hinshaw et al., 1979). At that time the technology, in terms of resolution, was unable to compete with optical microscopy, and in contrast to the complications associated with the preparation of biopsy samples from patients, the dissection of plant materials to allow their microscopic examination is straight-forward and inexpensive. As a result, the utility of developing a non-invasive approach was for a long time not recognized by the plant science community; furthermore, at that time, a number of technical issues surrounding the processing of plant tissue (see §3, below) discouraged exploration of the potential of MRI.

In the wake of technical improvements with respect to both MRI (Van As & van Duynhoven, 2013; Borisjuk et al., 2012) and experimental biology (Weissleder & Pittet (2008; Fiorani & Schurr, 2013), the scenario now looks quite different. The development of high throughput 'omics technology has produced large quantities of gene transcription, translation and post-translational data. Nevertheless, based as they generally are on invasive sampling, the reconstruction of *in vivo* processes from these data is difficult. Inevitably, destructive sampling can only give a snapshot of the condition of a once-living tissue, whereas the reality of the living organism is that conditions are in dynamic flux. Modelling has been used in an attempt to integrate 'omics data, but the predictive ability of any model is limited by the quality and breadth of the data used to construct it. The paradigm in much of the medical research field has shifted to non-destructive sampling, and in particular MRI. A similar transition in the plant sciences may be some way off, but is highly likely to occur in the coming years.

Plant tissues, just as those from all multicellular organisms, are inherently heterogeneous, and their global metabolism reflects the end result of a complex network of interactions between diverse cell types. During development and the adaptation to environmental cues or pathogen attack, changes in tissue structure are accompanied by many alterations in metabolism. Conventional histology in its many manifestations and state of art phenotyping (Fiorany & Schurr, 2013) is well suited for the identification of structural/functional alterations, but its resolving power for the spatial and/or temporal distribution of metabolites is very low. As a result, our understanding of most of the dynamic processes occurring in the plant cell, many of which are probably important for the determination of crop productivity, remains quite rudimentary.

Here, the aim is to convince the reader of the need to develop non-invasive approaches to study plant metabolism, and in particular to demonstrate the merits of MRI for this purpose. Some of the leading MRI-based strategies for metabolite imaging are explained, and the essential peculiarities of plant and animal (as an experimental models used for imaging) are highlighted. By concentrating on plants, we explore the opportunities offered, and the challenges posed by MRI for elucidating the metabolism of living organisms. We suggest that a co-operative effort between NMR physicists and plant biologists will yield a substantial research significant dividend.

1. Imaging Platforms Able to Visualize Metabolites

The imaging of the chemical composition of a tissue is typically a more challenging task than the visualization of its structure. A small number of potentially informative platforms have been suggested (Weissleder & Pittet, 2008, Aharoni & Brandizzi, 2012; Fiorani & Schurr, 2013). Here we summarize the most effective of such technologies: spatially resolved mass spectrometry imaging (MSI) and positron emission tomography (PET).

1.1. Mass Spectrometry in Spatially Resolved Mode

MSI is a relatively recent technology. It has the potential to determine the distribution of specific molecules in tissue sections via the use of direct ionization (McDonnel & Heeren, 2007; Lee et al., 2012). The choice of ionization source is significant when the subject is living tissue (IR frequency laser energy, for example, is more ablative than UV frequency). The level of spatial resolution achieved lies in the range 10–50 μm, with the new generation of MS devices able to produce a very high level of mass resolution and accuracy (Hu et al., 2005; Schaub et al., 2008). MSI is suited for the analysis of animal tissue sections (Khatib-Shahidi et al., 2006) and individual plant cells (Horn et al., 2012; Shrestha et al., 2009), and has found wide use for the *in situ* imaging of proteins, lipids, drugs and metabolites (Nimesh et al., 2013). In plant-based experiments, matrix-assisted laser desorption ionization (MALDI)–MSI has been successfully applied to map the metabolites present on the surface of *Arabidopsis thaliana* flowers and leaves (Jun et al., 2010), for the identification of the free fatty acids present at the surface of various fruits (Zhang et al., 2007), and to map the distribution of various lipids within the crop seeds (Horn et al., 2012). Although the capacity of conventional

MALDI to detect molecules smaller than 500 Da is limited, there is growing interest in using MALDI-MSI to characterize the content of small metabolites (Zhang et al., 2007; Wiseman et a., 2008; Cha et al., 2008). A description of and comparison between the various detection schemes employed to date, along with their potential for metabolite imaging have been reviewed elsewhere (Touboul et al., 2011; Gode et al., 2013).

A number of methodological improvements, as well as a range of "soft ionization" approaches for imaging intact molecules, are appearing in the literature. A general drawback of current MSI technology is that it is either limited to the analysis of the sample surface or requires extensive pre-preparation of the tissue. Kinetic MSI, perhaps the most advanced of current methods, while it provides quantifiable information regarding metabolic flux both spatially and temporally, still only provides clinicians with a picture of events at or near the sample surface or in sections (Louie et al., 2013). Several technical problems still limit the widespread application of MSI (Miura et al., 2012). The need to balance structural and chemical integrity with data quantification/validation remains a key issue for MSI, including the most advanced forms of the technology, such as laser ablation electrospray ionization (Shrestha et al., 2009), desorption electrospray ionization (Li et al., 2013; Müller et al., 2011) and nanostructure-initiator MS (Louie et al., 2013).

1.2. Positron Emission Tomography (PET)

PET utilizes radioactive nuclei to label biological molecules. Its spatial resolution is in the order of mm, and it can provide quantitative information regarding dynamic processes over a relatively large field of view. Like MRI, PET allows imaging through opaque tissue, even if the thickness of the sample is large (Köckenberger et al., 2004; Phelps, 2004). PET experiments in plants have achieved the necessary labelling by integrating short half-life positron-emitting isotopes into either metabolites, nutrients or water. The isotopes used to date have included ^{11}C (Minchin & Thorpe, 2003), ^{13}N (Ohtake et al., 2001; Kiyomiya et al., 2001), ^{15}O (Nakanishi et al., 2003) and ^{18}F (Kiyomiya et al., 2001; Nakanishi et al., 2003, Tanoi et al., 2005). While earlier radio-tracer based studies were only able to monitor metabolite transport and accumulation on a coarse spatial scale, PET-based ones have produced a much higher level of resolution (Keutgen et al., 2002). PET has also shown substantial potential for *in planta* analysis because of its high sensitivity (Babst et al., 2005; Jahnke et al., 2009). Since the spatial resolution of the ^{11}C assay is limited to ~1.3 mm

(Phelps et al., 1975; Streun et al., 2006, 2007), it is best suited to the characterization of long distance translocation (Schwachtje et al., 2006; de Schepper et al., 2013). Most recently, PET has been extended to observe real time variation in metabolite content (Beer et al., 2010; Alexoff et al., 2011; de Schepper et al., 2013). PET requires a complex system for imaging and co-registration (for example it can be coupled with MRI, see Jahnke et al., 2009). In this configuration, PET is used for the detection of the target metabolite(s), while MRI supplies the non-invasive visualization of the sample's internal structure.

MRI is less sensitive than PET (Metzler et al., 1995; Melkus et al., 2009b); given that they represent different modalities, data acquisition and processing are consequently rather complex (Bühler et al., 2011). A weakness of PET is that it is impossible to determine which specific molecule the decaying nucleus is associated with. Moreover, standard PET cannot be used for dual isotope imaging (which permits the simultaneous investigation of two different biological processes), because positron-electron annihilation products from different tracers are often indistinguishable from one another in terms of their energy output. Dual isotope PET requires that one of the two radioactive isotopes is a pure positron emitter and that the other emits additional high energy γ radiation (Andreyev & Celler, 2011). A further difficulty surrounds the health and safety aspects of using a strong positron emitter in a laboratory situation. A review of PET systems and their usage in plant research is given by Kiser et al. (2008).

PET systems have been in use in the medical field for over 30 years (Ter-Pergossian et al., 1975) and miniaturized instruments are deployed both in a number of experimental programmes and in clinical practice (Chatziioannou, 2002; Rohren et al., 2004). Combined PET–MRI methods have been experimented with to assess cardiac parameters in an infarct mouse model (Büscher et al., 2010), as well as to image the structure, function and molecular profile of brain tumors (Boss et al., 2010). A very recent application of PET has described the cellular mechanisms of certain diseases and some pharmaceutical consequences of specific treatments, leading to the novel notion that a specific cellular metabolic condition, rather than the presence of a distinct molecule(s), provides the most useful target for future anti-cancer therapies (Dörr et al., 2013). Generally, however, although PET provides an effective means for performing *in vivo* studies, its major limitation in the context of plant science is inadequate spatial resolution and, probably more significantly, its requirement for radioactive labelling for detection.

2. NMR-Based Tools and Applications

The theoretical basis of MRI has been described both for the reader with a strong background in physics (Callaghan, 1991; Haacke et al., 1999; de Graaf, 2007; McRobbie, 2006) and in versions more accessible to the biologist (Köckenberger et al., 2001, 2004; 2009; Elliot & Skerrit, 2006; Blümler et al., 2009). The content of this section covers the technical aspects of MRI for which an understanding is helpful to optimize experimental design in the area of metabolite imaging.

2.1. Choosing the Most Accessible Elements

MRI is based on the quantum mechanical property of nuclear spin. Nuclei containing an odd number of neutrons and an odd number of protons, as well as nuclei in which the sum of the number of neutrons and protons is odd, are associated with the non-zero net magnetic moment which allows them to be targeted by NMR. In a typical experiment, the sample is exposed to a strong main magnetic field (B_0) which forces an appropriate nucleus to align itself with the field. The resulting torque exerted by the field on the spinning nucleus induces a circular motion called precession. The frequency ϑ_0 of the precession (or the Larmor frequency) depends on the gyromagnetic ratio γ of the nucleus and is proportional to the external magnetic field: $\vartheta_0 = \gamma \cdot B_0/2\pi$. Among the biologically significant elements, H, C, N, O, F, Na and P are suitable for NMR. Together, this set of elements constitutes 99% of organic matter. A range of stable isotopes can be used, although in some cases there is a choice between different isotopes of a given element (e.g., ^1H and ^2H, ^{14}N and ^{15}N), provided that they have distinct inherent receptivity (Table 1). A single Larmor frequency for a certain nucleus would not be of interest in a metabolic study because the signal detected from this nucleus in the sample would be associated with a single frequency. Fortunately the molecular environment influences the magnetic field at the nucleus, leading to a small shift in its Larmor frequency, referred to as the “chemical shift”, and it is this feature which makes NMR interesting for metabolic studies. Different molecules can be detected and identified based on differences between their resonance frequencies (“NMR spectrum”). The NMR spectra of a range of metabolites are well documented, allowing MRI spectra to be treated as diagnostic identifiers of specific metabolites (de Graaf, 2007; Govindaraju et al., 2000).

Table 1. NMR properties of biological significant nuclei

Nucleus	Spin	Natural abundance [%]	γ[MHz/T]	Relative sensitivity	NMR frequency at 7.05T [MHz]
^{1}H	1/2	99.9	42.576	1.00	300.0
^{2}H	1	1.5x10-2	6.536	$1.45x10^{-6}$	46.1
^{13}C	1/2	1.1	10.71	$1.76x10^{-4}$	75.5
^{14}N	1	99.6	3.076	$1.00x10^{-3}$	21.7
^{15}N	1/2	3.7x10-1	-4.316	$3.86x10^{-6}$	30.4
^{17}O	5/2	3.7x10-2	-5.774	$1.08x10^{-5}$	40.7
^{19}F	1/2	100	40.054	0.83	282.2
^{23}Na	3/2	100	11.262	$9.27x10^{-2}$	79.4
^{31}P	1/2	100	17.235	$6.65x10^{-2}$	121.4

The ^{1}H nucleus is generally deemed to be highly sensitive and is therefore the isotope of choice in most *in vivo* NMR and MRI applications. It is a very abundant and stable nucleus in nature and its NMR spectrum is distinct from that of ^{2}H. Only disadvantage is that ^{2}H has negative effects on cell growth (Sacchi & Cocucci, 1992). ^{2}H can only be used in plant NMR experiments as a low concentration tracer (Link & Seelig, 1990), but has been useful in *in vivo* experiments to assess water movement in the eye (Obata et al., 1995) and blood flow (Furuya et al., 1997).

The ^{19}F nucleus has a high relative NMR sensitivity. While the abundance of fluorine in plants is low, xenobiotic compounds could be introduced into the organism to study transport or flux through a particular metabolic pathway or to measure the local pH (Ratcliffe & Roscher, 1998). However, ^{19}F NMR has not been widely used in plant research. Among the few examples of its use, a fluorinated compound and ^{19}F NMRI were used to study synthetic pathways in live plants of the species *Ancistrocladus heyneanus* (Bringmann et al., 2001). In contrast, ^{19}F NMR has enjoyed a long history of use in animal and human material (Chen et al., 2010). Prominent applications have been the imaging of gene expression based on tracers in the context of drug pharmacokinetics and metabolism (Lockhart et al., 1991; Litt, 1995; Ruiz-Cabello et al., 2011; Terekhov et al., 2013), measuring tissue oxygen status (Mason et al., 2003; Liu et al., 2011), pH (Huang et al., 2013) and inflammation (Waiczies et al., 2013; Balducci et al., 2013; Weibel et al., 2013).

The ^{13}C nucleus offers access to a wide range of metabolites, as effectively all metabolically relevant molecules are organic. Furthermore, ^{13}C

NMR spectra display sharp resonances over a wide chemical shift separation, which facilitates the identification of metabolites from their ^{13}C NMR spectra. The low natural abundance (1.1%) of the isotope makes it a difficult nucleus to be detected in *in vivo* NMR experiments (its relative detection sensitivity factor is 5700 fold less that than of ^{1}H (Table 1). This challenge is being tackled in various ways (see §4) (Heidenreich et al., 1998; Kalusche et al., 1999; Melkus et al., 2011). On the other hand, advantage can be taken of its low abundance to study the dynamic uptake and metabolism of ^{13}C labelled molecules, following feeding with exogenous ^{13}C labelled substrate (de Graaf et al., 2011; Rolletschek et al., 2011).

Among the N isotopes, ^{14}N is the more sensitive at its natural abundance, whereas ^{15}N yields much narrower NMR resonances. ^{14}N has a spin of I=1 and therefore an electric quadrupole moment which results in a more rapid relaxation times and broader line widths. The relative NMR sensitivity of the ^{15}N nucleus is 260,000 fold less than that of ^{1}H. In principle, ^{15}N can be employed for *in vivo* NMR, as well as for imaging, but various enhancement schemes have to be implemented to facilitate the acquisition of meaningful ^{15}N NMR data (Fox et al., 1992; Kanamori & Ross, 1999). To the best of our knowledge, no reported ^{15}N images of metabolites have been published.

The isotopes ^{23}Na and ^{31}P are sufficiently abundant in the human body to be detected directly. The feasibility of using ^{23}Na for the non-invasive monitoring of NaCl accumulation in plant seedlings was demonstrated by Olt et al. (2000), who achieved a spatial resolution of $156\times156\ \mu m^2$ and a temporal resolution of 85 min. Quantitative and qualitative ^{23}Na MRI of the human kidney has been reported by Haneder et al. (2011), while the dynamics of ^{23}Na concentration during tissue aging in humans has been described by Kopp et al. (2013). ^{23}Na has been exploited in various experiments to measure on intact plants (Olt et al., 2000) and animals (Neuberger et al., 2007; Jansen et al., 2004). The ^{31}P nucleus has an important advantage over that of ^{1}H (Moon & Richards, 1973), since the chemical shift (see §2.1) of the organic phosphate compound is dependent upon the local pH. Consequently, it is possible to use chemical shift as a proxy for pH *in vivo*. ^{31}P-based MRI can achieve a sub-millimeter level of resolution for pH, which is adequate for entomological subjects (Hugg et al., 1992; Skibbe et al., 1995; Hart et al., 2003). ^{31}P-based MRI has been used to visualize gene expression in animals (Gilad et al., 2008), so could presumably be used for a similar purpose in plant subjects (Borisjuk et al., 2012). Its disadvantage is the rather low sensitivity of ^{31}P.

The relatively low detection sensitivity and low abundance of the X-nuclei (^{13}C, ^{31}P and ^{15}N) in comparison to ^{1}H is a primary consideration in most applications. Low natural abundance can be considered to be an advantage because it allows position labelled compounds to be used to monitor the flux of labelled metabolites through a metabolic network (e.g. ^{13}C in carbohydrates or ^{15}N in amino acids). The need for a high strength magnetic field and specific radio frequency (RF) coils is a secondary, but potentially important consideration, especially when isotopes other than ^{1}H are being used.

2.2. Hardware Design (Magnets, Gradients and Resonators)

The majority of MRI-based investigations targeting metabolites have used relatively high magnetic field strengths which maximize the signal-to-noise ratio (SNR) (van As & van Duynhoven 2013). The strongest currently commercially available MRI microscope has a field strength of 21.1 T, which corresponds to a ^{1}H resonance frequency of 900 MHz, and represents an approximately seven fold greater field than is offered by routine clinical MRI scanners. The gain in sensitivity and the increased chemical shift dispersion obtained by increasing the magnetic field strength has encouraged the development of stronger superconducting magnets. Gradient coils are needed to encode the spatial localization of the spins; they are inserted into the magnet bore in order to create three orthogonal gradients in the magnetic field (Figure 1A-C). For clinical applications, the gradients are typically less than 100 mT/m, whereas those for pre-clinical applications range from 200 -600 mT/m, while for current vertical ultra high magnetic field MRI instruments, the range is 1-3 T/m. Such gradients are adequate for the *in vivo* scanning of small animal subjects (rodents). The rise-time of the gradient (i.e., the time needed for the gradient to be fully established), which is also an important parameter, can vary from >100 microseconds to several milliseconds.

The RF resonators act as antennae, and are adjusted to the sample in order to interact with the spin system by both producing the magnetic field (which excites the spin system) and detecting the response (Figure 1D-F). The resonator is tuned to the Larmor frequency of the nuclei to be detected. When imaging other nuclei, the shift in sensitivity of the NMR has to be considered and may require the creation of a corresponding single- or multi- resonant coil (see Table 1). Various coil/resonator configurations have experimented with the imaging of plant metabolites. Volume resonators produce a very homogeneous B_1 field (which is required for quantitative metabolite spectroscopy and imaging), but are generally less sensitive than surface coils.

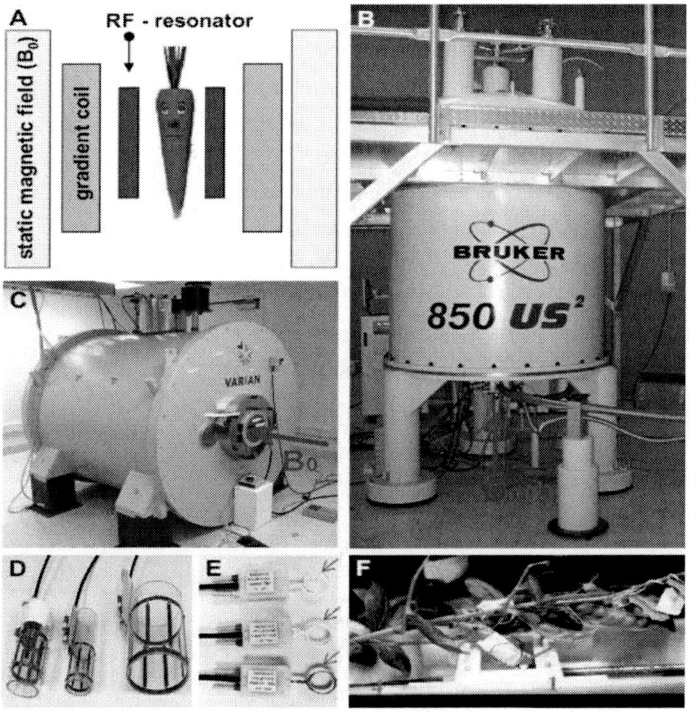

Figure 1. Principles of magnetic resonance and devices used for MR-imaging. (A) Schematic experimental setup for MRI experiments; carrot as example for the biological subject is positioned in the centre of the MRI instrument. The object is surround by the NMR coil (RF resonator), the gradients (gradient coil) and the static main magnetic field (B_0). (B) Ultra high field (20 Tesla, 850 MHz ^{1}H resonance frequency) NMR/MRI system with vertical bore operating with a 3 T/m gradient system; usable space: 1.9 cm inner diameter. The red arrow indicates the direction of the main magnetic field (B_0). (C) Pre-clinical MRI system with horizontal bore and a field strength of 7 Tesla (300 MHz ^{1}H resonance frequency). The inner diameter of the gradient system is 12 cm and the system typically used for pre-clinical *in vivo* rodent imaging. The red arrow indicates the direction of the main magnetic field (B_0). (D) Various volume (birdcage) resonators for ^{1}H imaging and localized spectroscopy: coils for mouse body, mouse head and rat body imaging (from left to right). (E) 2 cm diameter surface coils for: ^{1}H, ^{19}F (upper coil), ^{13}C, ^{15}N (middle coil) and ^{23}Na, ^{31}P (lower coil). The red arrows point to the actual NMR coil, which is the wired loop on the picture (F) NMR coil application for measurements on young pod of legumes: (1) position for climate chamber, (2) NMR coil, (3) joining wires (4) isolation tube. For further details see Borisjuk et al., 2012.

Some real examples include solenoids and scroll coils, which have an opening perpendicular to the direction of the main magnetic field and are therefore only practical for rather short samples such as the cereal grain (Neuberger et al., 2009a) and the tobacco seed (Fuchs et al., 2013); and birdcage coils and transverse electromagnetic resonators, in which the opening lies parallel to the magnetic field, so allowing for the imaging of relatively long samples, such as the barley spike (Figure 1D) (Melkus et al., 2011; Rolletschek et al., 2011). The most common surface resonators are single loop coils, which can be readily placed next to the target portion of the subject (Figure 1E). The sensitivity of surface resonators is usually much higher than that of volume resonators, but only the subject's surface can be imaged. The quantification process of the signal requires a signal correction step and an additional measurement of the coil sensitivity profile.

2.3. Advantages of Multinuclear Applications

Double nucleus (^{1}H and X) imaging requires transmitter/receiver coils capable of operating at two frequencies while maintaining good performance at each frequency. In multinuclear applications, the coil system generates and detects magnetic fields at at least two Larmor frequencies (double resonance NMR coils). For example, when detecting ^{1}H and ^{31}P using a 7.05 T magnet, the coils need to resonate at 300.0 MHz for ^{1}H and at 121.4 MHz for ^{31}P (Table 1). Combinations such as ^{1}H and ^{13}C (de Graaf et al., 2011), ^{1}H and ^{31}P (Klomp et al., 2011; Masad & Grant, 2011) and ^{1}H and ^{15}N (Kanamori & Ross, 1997) have all been successfully used. Since maximizing the sensitivity requires that the coil and the object be of comparable size, clinical coils or those used for rodent research are not well suited for investigating the metabolism of a crop seed. Commercial double resonant coils are available for human and animal MRI, but to the best of our knowledge, the coils needed for plant applications have all been custom-made to date.

Applications involving multi-nuclear *in vivo* MRI are generally primarily confined to research laboratories for now. However, combined imaging is of importance because it opens new possibilities for monitoring metabolism and gene expression in living tissue. In an experiment where a double resonant coil for the ^{1}H- and the X-nucleus is applied, the ^{1}H images can also be used to provide a highly detailed morphological image to go with the X-Nucleus metabolite maps, which typically have a lower spatial resolution. A further benefit of detecting the ^{1}H and X nuclei in the same experimental setup is that homogenization ("shimming") of the main magnetic field is eased, because the high SNR of the water-proton signal can be used for that procedure. In the authors' opinion, multinuclear imaging has the potential to revolutionize the evaluation of both the temporal and spatial profiles of gene expression and metabolism in living tissue.

3. Plant *vs.* Animal Models and Cautionary Notes for Using MRI

Plant and animal tissues share many similarities in terms of structure, composition and metabolism, but differ in many ways too. Hence protocols developed for animal/medical use cannot generally be directly applied to plant subjects. As an experimental subject, plants are more convenient than humans or animals because long exposures to NMR are clearly impossible in a clinical setting where the length of time a patient can remain still is limited. Even when animals are anaesthetized, exposure time can only be a maximum of a few hours. High magnetic field strengths are associated with enhanced sensitivity, but cognizance does needs to taken of the potential risk that they have an impact on living tissue (Formica & Silvestri, 2004; Paul et al., 2006). However, plants do not appear to be sensitive to either the noise generated by the machine, nor to strong magnetic fields (Osuga and Tatsuoka, 1999; Paul et al., 2006). This allows, for instance, the application of many, intense and very short excitation pulses. Thus MRI on plants can be performed in a much more direct and quantitative way than in humans (Blümler et al., 2009).

Unlike animal cells, the plant cell is bounded by a cellulose wall. While adjacent cells are interconnected via plasmodesmata, they are also separated from one another by air- or water-filled intracellular space. The presence of small, air-filled intercellular spaces can induce local heterogeneity in the magnetic field which can give rise to susceptibility artifacts (Callaghan et al., 1994; Connelly et al., 1987; Haacke & Liang, 2000). Further problems can arise when long term experiments are conducted. The trade-off is between the orientation and the bore diameter of the instrument. Most plants sense the direction of gravity, so the orientation of the main magnetic field needs to be vertical (Chudek & Hunter, 1997). While an animal/human MRI device is usually oriented horizontally (Figure 1C) with a bore diameter up to 60 cm, the diameter of a vertical bore for high field NMR systems (Figure 1B) equipped with the imaging gradients system can be as much as ten fold smaller, restricting its use to rather small subjects. For whole plant subjects, specific regions can be targeted by the judicious placement of RF resonators (Figure

1F), a measure which simultaneously enhances sensitivity and shortens the measurement time. The construction of such RF resonators can require technical innovation (Neuberger & Webb, 2009b).

Plants respire in the absence of light and photosynthesize in its presence. Unlike animal subjects, they cannot simply be fed before the experiment; instead, they need to be continuously supplied with water, nutrients and light. Customized controlled climate chambers have been devised with this in mind (van As, 2007). However, the internal space within an MRI device is restricted. A particularly innovative approach is represented by the design of split coil magnets which allowed the possibility of working with a larger subject although metabolite imaging may not feasible in this case because of the difficulty of imposing a high enough field strength and therefore sufficient SNR. Nevertheless, in some situations, a high degree of spatial resolution is not always necessary, as elaborated elsewhere (Köckenberger, 2001; van As et al., 2009; Borisjuk et al., 2013a).

4. Established NMR Techniques for Metabolite Imaging of Living Organisms

Theoretically, MRI can be used to detect and image the nuclei of almost any isotope of any element which has a nuclear magnetic moment other than zero. Hydrogen is the most commonly used element, because firstly ^{1}H has very high relative sensitivity compared to other nuclei, and secondly water (with its two ^{1}H atoms) is ubiquitous in biological tissues. While MRI generates highly resolved images of tissues by detecting the ^{1}H nuclei within the water molecule (i.e., it derives spatial information based on the nuclear spins of the water ^{1}H atoms), *in vivo* NMR spectroscopy techniques are able to differentiate between and to quantify more complex molecules. The main difference between detecting water and metabolites is their concentration in the subject. In biological tissues, water is highly abundant, while the concentration of typical metabolites is around five orders of magnitude less. Detecting the ^{1}H signal from a metabolite requires the suppression of the large signal produced by the water, otherwise the water resonance would swamp the signal and so prevent a clear detection of the metabolites (de Graaf, 2007).

Various techniques have been developed to suppress the water signal, most commonly relying on pre-saturation using spectral selective pulses (Haase et al., 1985; Tkác et al., 1999). In subsequent NMR spectrum acquisition experiments, the amplitude of the water resonance signal is greatly reduced or even removed. Metabolites are imaged at a much lower level of spatial resolution than water to achieve a sufficient SNR from each voxel. Thus, the requirements for the experimental setup, the quality of the send/receiver coil and the signal-detecting pipeline must be exceptionally fine to detect NMR metabolite signals. Its capacity to acquire both the water content (which allows high resolution morphological imaging) and metabolite localization makes MRI a powerful *in vivo* research tool.

Various localized *in vivo* NMR spectroscopy and spectroscopic MRI approaches have been developed over the last decades to preserve chemical shift information and simultaneously to provide local information or a spatial map. Single voxel spectroscopy (SVS) is one of these methods: it enables the acquisition of a NMR spectrum from a given localized voxel. A second approach, which acquires spectral and spatial information from multiple voxels at the same time, is referred to as chemical shift imaging (CSI). CSI typically generates three- (or four-) dimensional datasets, in which the NMR spectrum is the additional dimension on top of the two- (three)-dimensional spatial information. This technique offers the opportunity to visualize various metabolites in a single experiment. A third approach (chemical shift selective imaging) is based on two- or three-dimensional imaging to obtain high resolution images of particular chemical shift species under specific circumstances. These techniques allow for rapid imaging times and good spatial resolution provided that the concentration of the target metabolite is sufficiently high. If metabolite resonances overlap, two-dimensional spectroscopy methods can be applied to distinguished between the different signals.

These methods have been developed for the high resolution NMR spectroscopy of liquids and can be applied alongside localized spectroscopy or spectroscopic imaging methods. Spectral editing methods can be used to simplify the NMR spectrum in the case of overlapping resonances; these sequences focus typically on one particular metabolite which is obscured by co-resonant signals, avoiding the need to acquire a complete two-dimensional spectroscopic dataset.

4.1. Single Voxel Spectroscopy (SVS)

SVS methods enable the acquisition of an NMR spectrum for a defined location in the subject. Magnetic field gradients are used to localize the voxel where the NMR spectrum is to be sampled. Various techniques have been developed to ensure correct localization. The three leading methods are image selected *in vivo* spectroscopy (ISIS: Ordidge et al., 1986), stimulated echo acquisition mode (STEAM: Frahm et al., 1987) and point resolved spectroscopy (PRESS: Bottomley, 1984a). A PRESS-localized ^{1}H NMR spectrum from a 1x1x1 mm^3 voxel from the endosperm of a wild type pea seed is illustrated in Figure 2A. In addition to the suppressed signal from water (H_2O), resonances from various metabolites are detectable using this technique, allowing the levels of sucrose (Suc), alanine (Ala) and glutamine (Gln) to be quantified and monitored over time by repeating the experiment (Figure 2B,C).

Newer, more precise SVS techniques are emerging from the pre-clinical and medical field; for example, localization by adiabatic selective refocusing (LASER: Garwood & DelaBarre, 2001), frequency offset corrected inversion (FOCI: Kinchesh & Ordidge, 2005) and the use of shorter echo times for the acquisition of spectra (Tkác et al., 1999; Mlynárik et al., 2006). These developments will increasingly give access to the macromolecular content of the sample (using short echo times) and improve the SNR of the resonances. Such methods should be readily adaptable for the investigation of plant metabolism and the characterization of larger target molecules.

4.2. Chemical Shift Imaging (CSI)

CSI (also referred to as MRSI - magnetic resonance spectroscopic imaging) detects NMR spectra from the simultaneous sampling of several voxels, a feature which is helpful for imaging the distribution of metabolites (Brown et al., 1982).

The technique acquires both spatial and spectral information in the same experiment. Such three (one spectral and two spatial dimensions) or four (one spectral and three spatial dimensions) dimensional datasets capture a plethora of metabolite-associated information. CSI allows (i) the monitoring of more than one metabolite simultaneously, because the resonances of the various metabolites are distinct; (ii) the quantification of metabolites via calibration with reference compounds; and (iii) the possibility of observing the dynamic behavior of some metabolites.

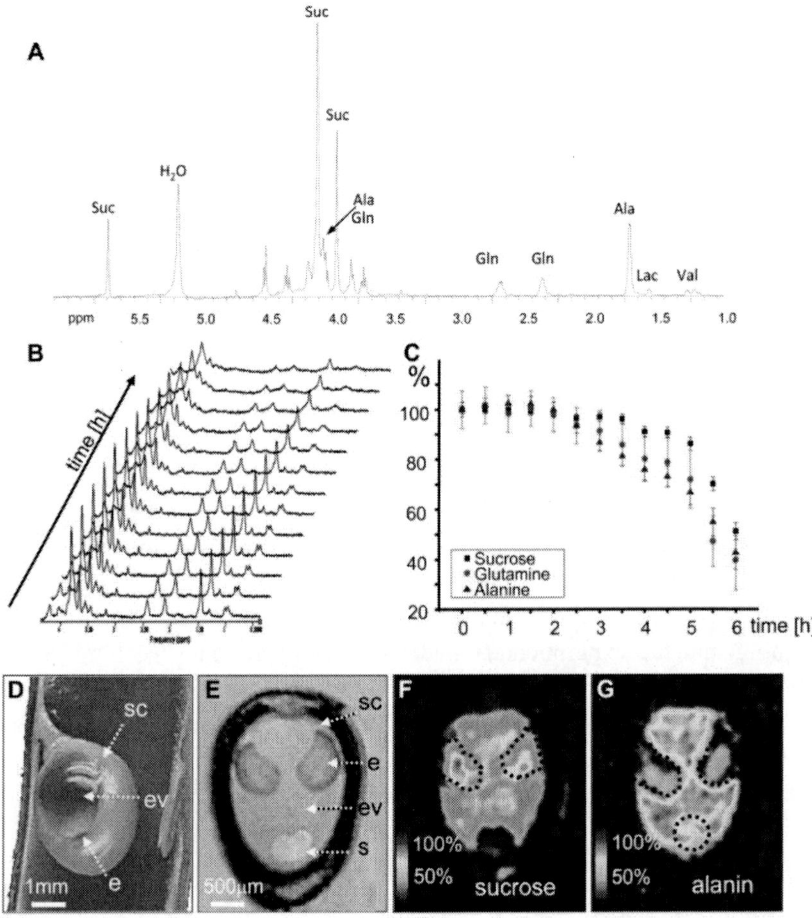

Figure 2. Localized ^{1}H NMR spectra and metabolic mapping of wild type pea seeds. (A) Localized ^{1}H NMR spectrum from the endosperm using PRESS: Besides residual signal from water (H_2O) resonances from the metabolites sucrose (Suc), alanine (Ala), glutamine (Gln), lactate (Lac) and valine (Val) are detectable. (B) Compositional changes of liquid endosperm during starvation: Localized NMR-spectra taken by monitoring of liquid endosperm of an individual seed (acquisition of localized NMR spectra in a 30 minutes interval). (C) Plot showing decline in the concentration of Suc, Gln and Ala during the starvation experiment; y-axis gives metabolite level in % (start of experiment is set to 100%). (D) Photo of the pea seed dissected per hand, liquid endosperm (correspond to endosperm vacuole (ev)), seed coat (sc) and embryo (e) are arrowed. (E) Visualisation of embryo sac by MRI shows positioning of seed coat (sc), embryo (e), endosperm vacuole (ev) and suspensor (s). (E) MRI visualisation of sucrose distribution within the embryo sac. Bar: color code for specific signal intensity. (F) Alanine distribution within the embryo sac. Bar represents color code for signal intensity. For further details see Melkus et al., 2009b.

Most of the metabolite CSI experimentation reported to date has relied on ^{1}H, ^{31}P, ^{23}Na and ^{13}C, although some users have successfully tested multi-resonant ^{19}F compounds as contrast agents. While the typical CSI experiment is rather time-consuming in comparison to MRI, it does offer a high level of sensitivity (Pohmann et al., 1997). Where the target is to image rapid metabolic changes, a number of methods have been derived to accelerate data acquisition (Pohmann et al., 1997). Thus, when multiple detection receiver coils are used (section §2.3), parallel imaging can be used to speed the acquisition of data (Dydak et al., 2003; Posse et al., 2013). Alternatively, compressed sensing (Hu et al., 2008; Kampf et al., 2010) can be exploited to reconstruct an under-sampled (and therefore more rapidly acquired) data set.

Clinical applications of CSI have largely been aimed at investigating metabolic changes in the human brain, although it has also had an impact in prostate and breast cancer research (Posse et al., 2013). CSI is commonly appended to a more extended MRI protocol, and so must be brief to minimize scan time and discomfort to the patient. The exposure time for a pre-clinical CSI experiment depends on how long the animal subject can safely be kept anaesthetized. Plant experiments can, in principle, be even more extended, assuming that the experimental conditions are appropriate (section §3). An early example is the imaging of lipids within the embryo of the pecan nut (Halloin et al., 1993). The spectra obtained from non-imbibed material contained a single major lipid peak, whereas those from imbibed embryos included separate water and lipid peaks. This separation enabled the distribution of both lipid and water to be determined. A further plant-based application involved the detection of sucrose in garden pea seed (Tse et al., 1996; Xia and Jelinski, 1995), fennel seed and the grape berry (Pope et al., 1991, 1993). ^{1}H CSI was used by Glidewell et al. (2002) to determine the distribution of water, sugars and lipids in the female cones of the conifer Afrocarpus falcatus. Some further examples of lipid imaging in plants using CSI have been summarized by Halloin et al. (1993) and Borisjuk et al. (2013a). The location of sugars in barley seeds during germination was investigated by Ishida et al. (1996). A representation of the distribution of sucrose and alanine within the endosperm of a garden pea seed is given in (Figure 2). Similarly, but using an inverse $^{13}C/^{1}H$ CSI method, the uptake into the barley caryopsis of ^{13}C enriched sucrose allowed the detection of sucrose (Figure 3) and its the metabolic products, in particular alanine (Figure 4). A pre-clinical application of using CSI in cancer research for *in vivo* investigation of the metabolic status of a xenograft tumor transplanted on the mouse leg is shown in Figure 5.

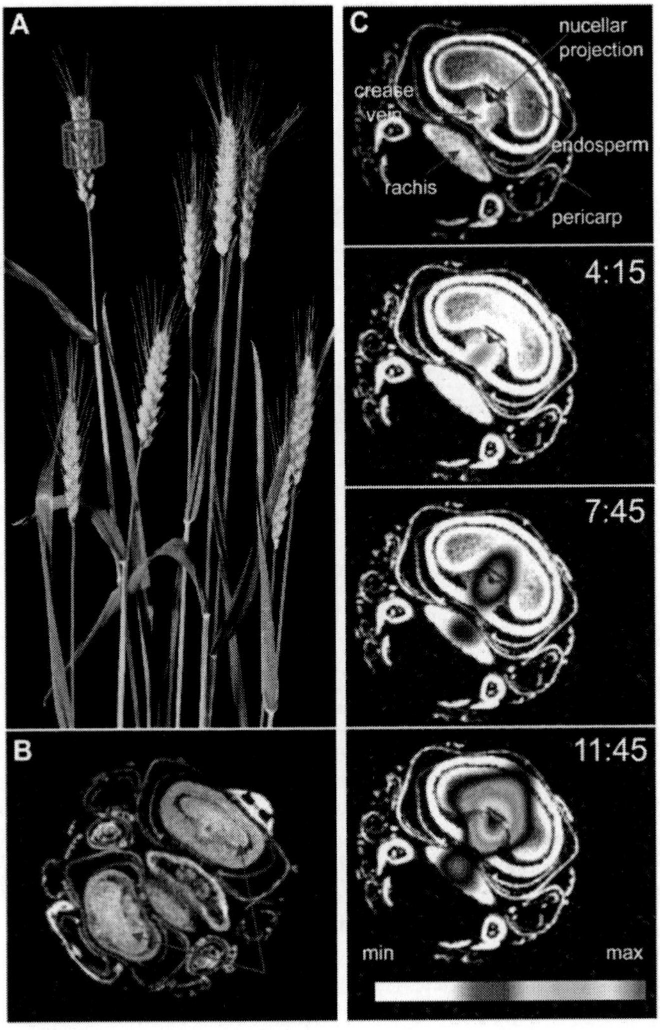

Figure 3. Non- invasive $^{13}C/^{1}H$ NMR imaging of ^{13}C sucrose allocation within the developing caryopsis of barley (*Hordeum vulgare*). (A) Young barley plant caring ears. The accumulation of ^{13}C in the barley caryopsis was performed during feeding a 100 mM ^{13}C labeled sucrose buffer solution to the stem. The red cage (schema) shows the position of the NMR coil. (B) A ^{1}H MRI image shows a cross section through the intact ear, two caryopses are visible (red arrows). (C) Fragments of the dynamic ^{13}C sucrose uptake imaging experiment: The reference image is shown at the top, below are samples of the color-coded ^{13}C sucrose maps at different time points demonstrating the uptake and distribution of ^{13}C sucrose. The time post the start of incubation is indicated on the upper right of each image (given in hours : minutes). For further details see Melkus et al., 2011.

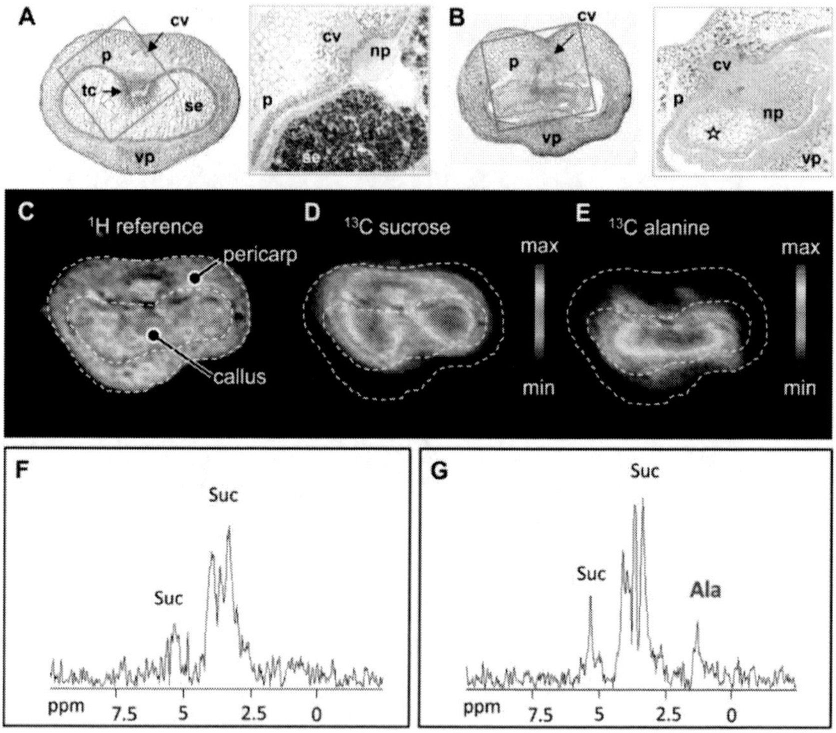

Figure 4. ^{13}C metabolic imaging of sucrose and alanine in barley seeds (*Hordeum vulgare*) using an inverse $^{13}C/^{1}H$ detection scheme (geHMQC). (A) The structure of the crease region of a wild type caryopsis, cross section. Nucellar projection is shown in green and starch accumulation as visualized by iodine staining in a wild type caryopsis (right). Dark staining visualizes starch accumulation, which is maximal in endosperm and absent in nucellar projection. (B) The structure of the crease region in *Jekyll* down-regulated line 91, cross section. Disordered nucellar projection is shown in green and starch accumulation as visualized by iodine staining in *Jekyll* down-regulated caryopsis. Endosperm is almost replaced by nucellar projection, which is asymmetrically vacuolized. (C) ^{1}H MR reference image of the *Jekyll* caryopsis. (D) Allocation of ^{13}C sucrose after 12h of feeding with a 100mM ^{13}C labelled sucrose buffer solution. (E) Alanine distribution after 12h of feeding with the 100mM ^{13}C labelled sucrose buffer solution. (F) Localized geHMQC $^{13}C/^{1}H$ spectrum from the pericarp region. The typical resonances from the ^{13}C labelled sucrose (Suc) are detectable. (G) geHMQC $^{13}C/^{1}H$ spectrum from the endosperm. Besides the resonances from ^{13}C sucrose also ^{13}C alanine (Ala) metabolized from the ^{13}C sucrose is visible. Abbreviations: cv, crease vein; np, nucellar projection; p, pericarp; se, starchy endosperm. For further details see Rolletschek et al., 2011.

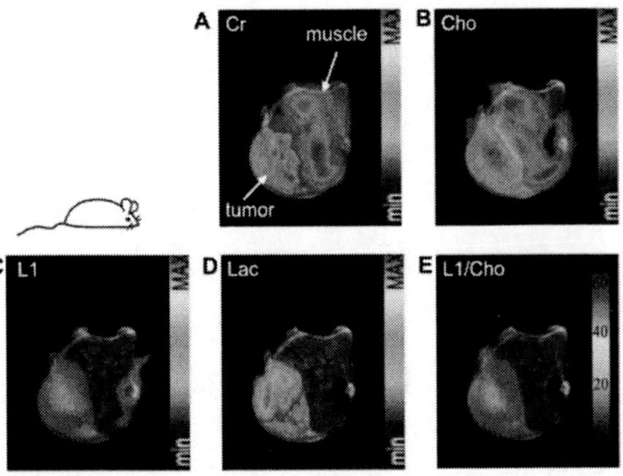

Figure 5. [1]H CSI metabolic imaging of a xenograft (SAS) tumor transplanted on the upper leg of a nude-mouse. (A-D) Interpolated metabolite maps acquired with CSI combined with Spectral Editing for lactate detection. The metabolite signal intensity is shown as color coded map over the ^{1}H reference image: (A) creatine (Cr), (B) choline-containing compounds (Cho), (C) lipid methylene groups (L1), (D) lactate (Lac). (E) The L1/Cho ratio map from the lipid L1 signal and the choline-containing compound. Large L1/ Cho ratios, originating from subcutaneous adipose tissue between skin and muscle, are omitted from the map. For further details see Melkus et al., 2008.

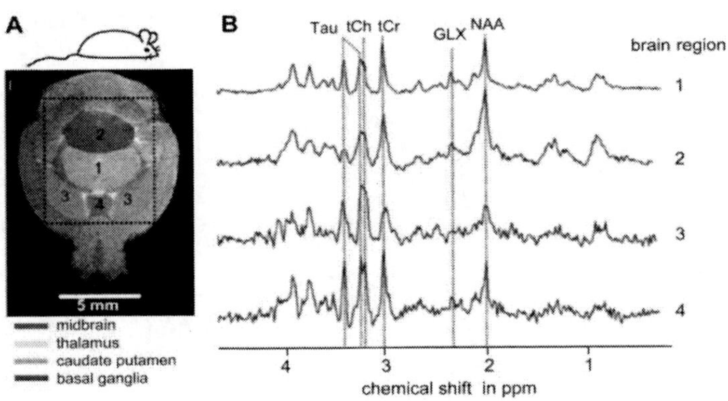

Figure 6. Visualization of metabolic heterogeneity of the mouse brain 20 days after date of birth using CSI (acquired at 17.6 Tesla). (A) Analyzed regions in the mouse brain: thalamus (region 1, yellow), midbrain (region 2, blue), caudate putamen (region 3, green) and basal ganglia (region 4, red). (B) *In vivo* spectra from the four mouse brain regions. Differences in the concentration of taurine (Tau) and N-acetylaspartate (NAA) between the brain regions were directly visible. Abbreviations: tCho, total choline; tCr, total creatine; GLX, glutamate and glutamine. For further details see Weiss et al., 2009.

The metabolites creatin, choline and lactate as well as mobiles lipids could be detected (Melkus et al. 2008). In a study by Weiss et al. (2009) CSI was used to acquire the ^{1}H NMR spectral pattern in different regions of the developing mouse brain using a main magnetic field strength of 17.6 Tesla (Figure 6).

4.3. Chemical Shift Selective Imaging

The acquisition of CSI data in two or three spatial dimensions is too unwieldy in certain experimental situations. Where the interest is focused on just a single metabolite or resonance frequency, it is possible to accelerate the experiment using frequency-selective excitation and/or refocusing (Bottomley, 1984b). Frequency-selective pulses are designed to specifically excite only a certain segment of the NMR spectrum, after which standard MRI is used to capture the signal. This approach is particularly useful when the metabolite's resonance is well separated from that of other compounds in the NMR spectrum. The visualization of lipids in biological samples is a good example of chemical shift selective imaging, since lipid resonances are well separated from that of water, and so lipids can readily be excited and/or refocused using spectral selective pulses (Figure 7).

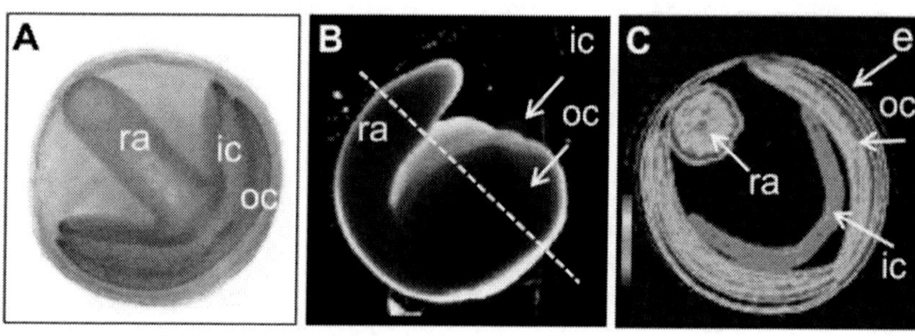

Figure 7. Lipid visualization in oilseed rape seed: conventional staining versus chemical shift selective MR-imaging. (A) Seed dissected at early storage stages, showing the seed coat and embryo inside of seed. (B) Embryos isolated at the same stage, showing the lipid distribution as visualized by conventional staining (Sudan III/IV dyes). (C) Intact seed at the same stage, showing the gradients in the lipid distribution (quantitative lipid map, max (red) 47µmol/g). For lipid MRI a chemical shift selective preparation with a standard multi-slice spin echo acquisition was used. Abbreviations: co, cotyledon; ic, inner cotyledon; oc, outer cotyledon; ra, radicle. For further details see Borisjuk et al., 2013.

Borisjuk et al. (2013a) have shown that this approach works well for imaging the lipid content of seeds and fruits. Various field strengths have proven to be effective, ranging from 4.7 T (Pope et al., 1991; Gussoni et al., 2001; Brescia et al., 2007) to 8.5 T (Terskikh et al., 2005) to 17.6 T (Neuberger et al., 2009a; Horn et al., 2012; Borisjuk et al., 2013a). Spatial (in plane) resolution can be as low as 25 μm (Gersbach & Reddy, 2002). Chemical shift selective imaging requires a highly homogeneous main magnetic field, otherwise artefactual results can arise, leading to false estimates of metabolite content. This is guaranteed by including shimming routines.

4.4. Localized Two Dimensional Spectroscopy

Metabolites which are difficult to identify in the NMR spectrum due to signal overlapping can sometimes be separated by adopting a two dimensional NMR approach, where the second dimension is created by additional scans which manipulate the spin system with additional RF pulses (Levitt, 2008). Correlation spectroscopy (COSY) is a basic two dimensional NMR spectroscopy method, where the chemical shift and the connection between neighboring nuclei in the molecule is visualized as so-called "cross peaks" in the 2D NMR spectrum. Two dimensional NMR can be combined with SVS (Thomas et al., 2001, 2003), as well as being capable of being built into CSI to enable the acquisition of a spatial map, in a combined technique referred to as correlation peak imaging (CPI) (Metzler et al., 1995; Ziegler et al., 1996; von Kienlin et al., 2000). Where the identity of most of the metabolites to be detected is known a priori, two dimensional techniques can help differentiate between signals which overlap in a simple one dimensional spectrum. For example, aspartate and phosphoethanolamine could be identified in the rat brain via cross peaks (von Kienlin et al., 2000). For metabolic studies performed on plant subjects, the expectation is that spectral overlaps will occur because of the presence of sucrose, glucose and fructose, and of various amino acids. The overlap is likely to be much stronger in *in vivo* than in *in vitro* subjects due to line broadening of the resonances. Figure 8 demonstrates an example of localized COSY applied to investigate the composition of sugars and amino acids in the endosperm of an intact garden pea seed; the cross peaks involving sugars and amino acids were readily resolved by implementing a second spectral dimension.

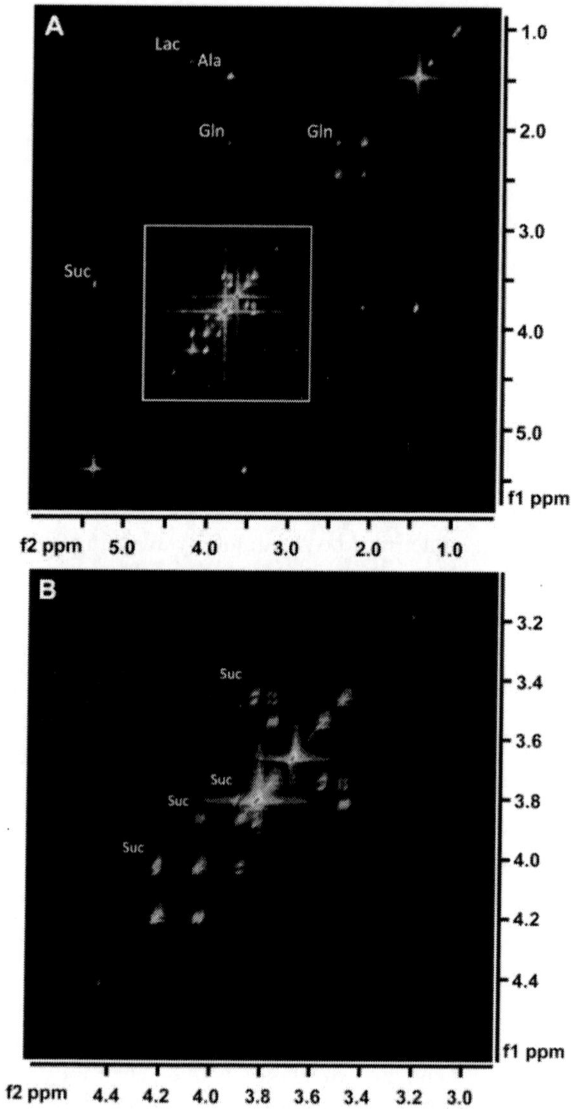

Figure 8. Localized two-dimensional NMR spectrum from the endosperm of wild type pea seeds (*Pisum sativum*). (A) Localized COSY (L-COSY) spectrum. The cross-peaks in the spectrum are indicated by the metabolite name labeling: Lac, lactate; Ala, alanine; Suc, sucrose. The white rectangle indicates the enlarged spectrum, which is presented in (B). (B) Enlarged spectrum from the white rectangle in (A). The cross-peaks detected between 3.2 ppm to 4.2 ppm result from sucrose. No other metabolites were detected in this spectral area. For further details see Melkus et al., 2009b.

A disadvantage of localized two dimensional NMR methods is their long acquisition time. Depending on the spectral resolution required and the bandwidth needed for the second (the indirect) spectral dimension, scan time is typically extended by a factor between 32 and 64 for *in vivo* scans. However, acceleration is possible, as referred to in section §4.2. The advantage and power of this approach is that a complete spectral pattern of the detectable metabolites is acquired, so allowing their discrimination from otherwise confounding metabolites.

4.5. Spectral Editing

The problem with the long acquisition times required in CPI and localized two dimensional NMR methods can be solved by spectral editing, but at a cost of losing some of the spectral information. Spectral editing methods are useful either when only a certain metabolite is of interest and/or when signal overlap is a problem.

Current methods rely on either polarization transfer (Hardy & Dumoulin, 1987), multiple quantum coherences (Sotak & Freeman, 1988) or the J-difference (Rothman et al., 1984) method to separate the target signal from co-resonant peaks.

The basics of these techniques have been presented by de Graaf (2007) and a description is beyond the scope of this chapter. Two acquisitions are necessary for J-difference spectroscopy, but the multi-quantum coherence approach requires only a single acquisition, as use is made of gradient de-phasing to unpick the overlapping signal.

A typical example of the successful implementation of spectral editing is the detection of lactate resonance in a background mass of mobile lipid signals. Figure 9 shows lactate images from a xenograft tumor transplanted on a mouse leg. The data was acquired using a spectral editing preparation in combination a standard CSI (Figure 9 A, B) and with a readout gradient method (Figure 9C) (Melkus et al., 2009a).

The significance of the level of lactate in a tumor has driven the development of various spectral editing methods (He et al., 1995; Smith et al., 2008; Boer et al., 2013). Wolf et al. (2000) used a double quantum filter combined with CSI to detect and image sucrose in the stem of sugar cane (*Saccharum officinarum*).

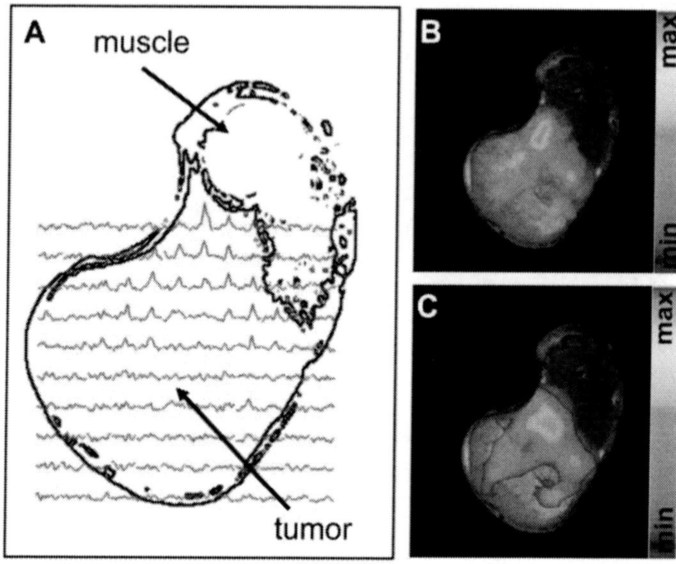

Figure 9. *In vivo* measurements of the lactate distribution in a xenograft (FADU) tumor transplanted on the upper leg of a nude-mouse using a spectral edited fast CSI sequence. (A) A spectral map of the edited lactate CH_3 resonance acquired with a spectral edited CSI sequence is laid over the tumor and leg contours. (B) The corresponding interpolated lacate distribution. (C) The interpolated lactate image acquired with the spectral edited fast CSI method. Both images were acquired in the same total measurement time to compare their sensitivities. For further details see Melkus et al., 2009a.

4.6. Considerations Surrounding NMR Metabolic Imaging

MRI is often the method of choice for assessing metabolite content and for monitoring metabolic reactions *in vivo* (Befroy, 2011; Befroy & Shulman, 2011). Its disadvantages are its relatively poor sensitivity and its requirement for sophisticated (and hence costly) equipment. A number of further considerations mitigating against the broad application of MRI in experimental biology are discussed later in this section. The resolving capacity of NMR improves with the strength of the main magnetic field, since this increases the SNR, while simultaneously enhancing the chemical shift separation. Unfortunately, it also raises the frequency of artefacts (Köckenberger, 2001), some of which result from the direct impact of high field strength on living cells (section §3). A validation procedure is therefore indicated, to ensure that metabolite concentrations measured non-invasively by MRI agree well with those derived from conventional destructive assays. The potential of localized NMR in biological research is high, but each of the current methods is associated with certain drawbacks. The technical operation of an NMR scanner is not a trivial procedure, few imaging protocols dedicated to plant subjects have so far been elaborated, and a level of fundamental understanding of the science underlying MRI is required to interpret the resulting data.

5. Implementation of Functional MRI in Experimental Plant Biology/Biotechnology

Plants (mostly their seed) are used as a vehicle to produce oil, proteins and a range of other valuable compounds. The overarching objective of crop genetic research is to engineer plant metabolism toward human needs. The focus of metabolic engineering efforts has shifted from manipulating single pathways to more holistic approaches, facilitated by high throughput 'omics technology (Yoon et al., 2013). Some of the most innovative plant MRI applications are being performed on crop species, rather than on model plants, with the driver being that a better understanding of how plant growth and metabolism are integrated during development and during adaptation to environmental cues and stresses will guide the design of novel or improved crops. Some examples follow which illustrate the role which MRI can play in these integrative approaches.

Example #1: Allocation of nutrients within the seed

In the plant, there is no vascular connection between the embryo and the mother plant. Attempts to characterize the connection using microscopy, laser dissection, isotope tracing and transgenesis have all failed to generate a complete picture. MRI, however, has succeeded in obtaining dynamic images of sucrose passing through the seed coat of species, then moving through a very small aperture into the interior of the seed. At the same time MRI was also able to visualize the amino acids synthesized from sucrose just after its entry into the storage tissue (Figure 4). An analysis of various mutant and transgenic barley lines has demonstrated that sucrose release via the nucellar projection provides an essential means whereby the mother plant controls the growth of the daughter caryopsis (Melkus et al., 2011). The distribution of the incoming sucrose was facilitated by the structural and metabolic features of the endosperm, leading to an *in silico* flux balance analysis of sucrose. None of this information was derivable using a conventional destructive approach.

Re-designing "functional MRI" (Köckenberger et al., 2004; Friis et al., 2007) to fit a seed subject has proven to be technically rather challenging. Solutes move within the plant vasculature quite slowly (Mullendore et al., 2010), and the speed of their dispersal outside the vasculature is expected to be slower still (Jenner et al., 1988; Patrick & Offler, 2001). Measuring solute movement with MRI is difficult when the flow velocity is in the order of 1 m/h or below, because of the need for strong MRI gradients which are applied for a long duration induce significant SNR loss (van As, 2007; Szimtenings et al., 2003). To surmount this problem, direct and inverse ^{13}C detection methods (such as the geHMQC sequence (Hurd & John, 1991)) to detect ^{13}C labelled tracers molecules have been combined with an optimized double resonant detector coil and a high magnetic field strength. The resulting metabolic images could be captured over about one hour for the direct ^{13}C measurements, and over 30 minutes for the inverse detection scheme. The required spatial scale for assaying a seed was a few millimeters, which allowed the ^{13}C NMR method to achieve a sufficient level of resolution within a reasonable measurement period. The method not only detected ^{13}C labelled sucrose, but also could identify other labelled metabolites (e.g. ^{13}C alanine). Finally, the $^{13}C/^{1}H$ NMR method allowed for a straightforward superimposition of the structural and the metabolite images, so enabling a precise localization of the metabolites within the subject.

Example #2: Potentially improved estimation of seed lipid concentration.

The capacity of individual tissues to accumulate lipids is hard to measure using conventional methods, which yield the mean concentration over a complete organ, rather than a localized one in a specific segment of the organ. The grain of barley, for example, not renowned as an oil crop, contains a mean lipid concentration of 2%, but MRI analysis has demonstrated that this concentration can exceed 50% in certain parts of the caryopsis, a level which matches that of genuine lipid crops (Neuberger et al., 2008, 2009a). MRI's ability to identify regions where lipids are either accumulated or degraded has allowed a more focused search for genetic variation with respect to lipid storage, as well as providing a tool to evaluate the response of the storage tissues to changes in the growing environment. MRI-based lipid mapping has been carried out on both very large (coconut) and very small (tobacco) seeds (Fuchs et al., 2013). Some of the ^{1}H MRI-based strategies described in sections §4.2 and §4.3 can be adapted to provide a quantification of lipids at very high levels of resolution (Neuberger et al., 2009a; Borisjuk et al., 2013a).

Example #3: Structural-functional alterations in storage product accumulation in a growing seed.

Oilseed rape, the leading European oilseed crop, has been a widely used model for studying the physiology and genetics of lipid synthesis and accumulation. However, both its seed size and embryo lipid content (which represents ~50% of seed dry weight) are in need of improvement to guarantee its continuing economic viability. The development of the embryo within the seed is difficult to follow using an invasive method, which is almost certain to disturb the process. After adjusting the MRI protocol to allow the imaging of small seeds, it has been possible to image aspects of seed metabolism and the development of lipid storage in the growing embryo, and to relate these to overall seed development. Such data were acquired by integrating ^{1}H MRI-based structural imaging with quantitative NMR-based visualization of lipids, supported by metabolic modelling and conventional analytical measurement of proteins, metabolites and enzymatic activity. The MRI platform used was a 17.6 T Avance II (Bruker, Rheinstetten, Germany) wide-bore system, implementing a multi-slice spin echo sequence with the water signal removed using a chemically selective suppression module. The sequence achieved an in-plane resolution of up to 20 μm isotropic and a slice thickness of 105 μm. The major finding was that the environment within the seed is heterogeneous due to the folding of the cotyledons, and that this generated localized variation in metabolic activity which resulted in distinct profiles of metabolites and storage products. The sessile nature of plants means that they must be able to adapt their metabolism to prevailing conditions of illumination, nutrition and physical space. For a detailed description, see Borisjuk et al. (2013), Schiebold et al. (2011) and Verboven et al. (2013).

The direct or indirect consumption of seed/grain is an important component of the human diet. Understanding how proteins, lipids, carbohydrates are accumulated in the seed, and then how they are digested in the human gut is important, not just for the purpose of improving crop productivity but also to find ways to overcome a number of human diseases. The potential contribution of MRI to food quality control has been noted. As early as 1994, Hisa et al. generated a MRI image of a nut lodged in the throat of a young boy, but it was some years before it became possible to image seed digestion in the human gut (Hoad et al., 2008). A subsequent evaluation of lipid digestion and absorption (Hoad et al., 2011) was able to provide a number of avenues for the design of foods with positive health benefits. Overall, it is clear that non-invasive MRI represents a versatile platform for the study of both plant and animal metabolism, of the fate of various nutrients in the human/animal gut, and should play a part in the diagnosis and alleviation of a number of food-related disorders.

6. Leading Edge MRI Applications in Animal/Medical Science and Prospects for Its Use in Plants

MRI technology and sequence development is, like most of the biotechnology field, led by developments in medical science. The investigation of metabolism is a fast developing research area, particularly in the context of animal models for potential translation to human subjects. Here we describe the three most recent innovations made in MRI, all of which could have considerable potential for application in the plant sciences.

Hyperpolarized ^{13}C MRI has been elaborated to monitor the uptake and metabolism of endogenous compounds. The hyperpolarization of the ^{13}C nucleus enables a gain in signal strength of between four and five orders of magnitude (Ardenkjaer-Larsen et al., 2003; Golman et al., 2006a). Methods to maintaining dynamic nuclear polarization in solution enables access to hyperpolarized contrast agents for MRI. The technique has been pioneered in various pre-clinical experiments, and especially as a tool to understand tumor metabolism (Golman et al., 2006b; Chen et al., 2007; Day et al., 2007; Gallagher et al., 2011), as well as in a range of other medical and biological contexts (Aquaro et al., 2013; Lau et al., 2013). A very recent report describes its use in an *in vivo* study of human subjects (Nelson et al., 2013); here, hyperpolarized [1-^{13}C] pyruvate was used to image metabolism in tumors of prostate cancer patients, and it was possible to show that local elevated [1-^{13}C] lactate [1-^{13}C] pyruvate ratios were diagnostic for tissue regions where a biopsy had indicated the presence of cancerous growth. The degree of the polarization shown by the metabolite, its ^{13}C T1 relaxation time and the time elapsed between hyperpolarization and the arrival of the metabolite at its target are all critical parameters which help to achieve the large gain in the SNR (Nelson et al., 2013). Once the hyperpolarized labelled metabolite has been produced, the ^{13}C signal decays rapidly (within a few seconds to several minutes, depending on the actual metabolite) due to T1 relaxation. For example, [1-^{13}C] pyruvate, a very commonly used analyte in cancer research, has a T1 relaxation time of one minute at 3 Tesla. Such short T1 relaxation times would represent a major disadvantage in any plant study, so novel strategies will need to be elaborated to lengthen relaxation time to allow the analyte sufficient time to reach its target tissue; alternatively, ways will need to be found to deliver the analyte directly to the site where metabolism is under study. As noted in section §3, plant cell structure differs greatly from that of a mammalian cell (particularly with respect to the existence of a thick cell wall), and this has consequences for the application of a technique such as hyperpolarized ^{13}C. Medical researchers are already focusing on hyperpolarizing other metabolically active compounds and also on using nuclei other than ^{13}C (Cudalbu et al., 2010; Cerutti et al., 2011).

A second promising MRI innovation involves imaging tissue using very short T2 relaxation times. Neither bones nor teeth are directly visible in classical MRI images, appearing only as dark regions. Both of these structures are characterized by very short T2 relaxation times, which has prevented the capture of signal from the protons present within them. Developments in hard- and software have enabled ultra-short echo time (UTE) sequences to be run on commercially available clinical MRI scanners (Gatehouse & Bydder, 2003). These methods are in current use to investigate bone and the bone-cartilage interface (Togao et al., 2010). The same approach has also been effective with lung tissue, since the contact of the lung with oxygen shortens the relaxation time and hence results in rapid signal decay. Sweep imaging with Fourier transformation (SWIFT) imaging uses an echo time close to zero (Idiyatullin et al., 2006). This approach has allowed for the direct imaging of teeth (Idiyatullin et al., 2011) and its success with imaging the bone-cartilage interface on equine specimens indicates its potential in musculoskeletal research (Rautiainen et al., 2013). Zero echo time (ZTE) imaging is a third type of sequence able to capture the signal when T2 times are short (Weiger et al., 2011). In dense and woody plant tissues, T2 relaxation times are expected to be short, so techniques such as SWIFT and ZTE will be needed to acquire the signal. Spectral selective water suppression could be combined with these techniques to image the lipid content of seeds, whose T2 relaxation times are too short for standard MRI methods. UTE, SWIFT and ZTE have the potential to enable a range of presently impractical non-invasive explorations of plants and seeds. For translation from animal/human to plant subjects, the development of new NMR coils may be necessary. Note that the acquisition of signal with ultra-short or close to zero echo times may risk capturing artefactual signals from the coil housing or the isolation material of the RF cable.

"MRI fingerprinting" has the capacity to extract various quantitative parameters (T1 relaxation time, T2 relaxation time, proton-density and off-resonance) using a sequence comprised of semi-random pulses and acquisition parameters (Ma et al., 2013). The acquired data results in a very specific fingerprint and is compared to a database of possible patterns. With this approach different quantitative maps can be reconstructed from the dataset. The new concept could have also several applications in plant imaging, as for example the quantitative imaging of lipids and metabolites, where the knowledge of T1 and T2 times are necessary for signal correction and quantification.

The step from animal to human MRI application has generally been rapid. The translation from animal/human to plants is more difficult, since typically it is not possible to replicate the same technique due to the major biological difference between animal and plant physiology and morphology. Generally, adjustments need to made to both the software and the hardware, along with the development of appropriate pre-MRI experimental procedures.

Conclusion

MRI has major potential as a platform to non-invasively analyze metabolism in living organisms. Its usage in plant research lags far behind that in medical research, and a substantial effort will be required both to enhance the levels of chemical and spatial resolution achievable and to re-design some of the hardware before its potential can be fully realized in plant research. Consideration needs to be given to ways in which the expense of using MRI facilities can be reduced to make the platform more accessible for the plant biologist. Despite the undoubted versatility of MRI, it cannot fully replace any of the other conventional high resolution and/or high throughput technologies. Indeed, the full explanatory power of MRI can only be achieved when it is coupled with high throughput 'omics technology and analytical and computational methods. The integration of imaging and 'omics data has become an important topic, as this is now required to form a more holistic view of the living organism. Visualization of *in vivo* processes may well have an impact on the interpretation of some molecular and biochemical data sets, helping to formulate rational mechanistic models and to understand what can seem to be uninterpretable results. MRI's major contribution to our understanding of life processes is that unlike in silico models it is based on real data; and unlike analyses based on destructive sampling, it is a non-invasive method which is less liable to produce artefactual data.

References

Aharoni, A & Brandizzi, F. (2012). High-Resolution Measurements in Plant Biology. *Plant J.,* 70: 1-4.

Alexoff, DL; Dewey, SL; Vaska, P; Krishnamoorthy, S; Ferrieri, R; Schueller, M; Schlyer, DJ; Fowler, J S. (2011). PET imaging of thin objects: measuring the effects of positron range and partial-volume averaging in the leaf of Nicotiana tabacum. *Nucl. Med. Biol.*, 38: 191-200.

Andreyev, A & Celler, A. (2011). Dual-isotope PET using positron-gamma emitters. *Phys. Med. Biol.*, 56: 4539-4556.

Aquaro, GD; Frijia, F; Positano, V; Menichetti, L; Santarelli, MF; Ardenkjaer-Larsen, JH; Wiesinger, F; Lionetti, V; Romano, SL; Bianchi, G et al. (2013). 3D CMR mapping of metabolism by hyperpolarized 13C-pyruvate in ischemia-reperfusion. *JACC Cardiovasc. Imaging*, 6: 743-744.

Ardenkjaer-Larsen, JH; Fridlund, B; Gram, A; Hansson, G; Hansson, L; Lerche, MH; Servin, R; Thaning, M and Golman, K. (2003). Increase in signal-to-noise ratio of > 10,000 times in liquid-state NMR. *Proc. Natl. Acad. Sci. USA*, 100: 10158-10163.

Babst, AB; Ferrieri, RA; Gray, DW; Lerdau, M; Schlyer, DJ; Schueller, M; Thorpe, MR; Orians, CM. (2005). Jasmonic acid induces rapid changes in carbon transport and partitioning in Populus. *New Phytol.*, 167: 63-72.

Balducci, A; Wen, Y; Zhang, Y; Helfer, BM; Hitchens, TK; Meng, WS; Wesa, AK and Janjic, JM. (2013). A novel probe for the non-invasive detection of tumor-associated inflammation. *Oncoimmunology*, 2: e23034.

Beer, S; Streun, M; Hombach, T; Buehler, J; Jahnke, S; Khodaverdi, M; Larue, H; Minwuyelet, S; Parl, C; Roeb, G; Schurr, U; Ziemons, K. (2010). Design and initial performance of PlanTIS: a high-resolution positron emission tomograph for plants. *Phys. Med. Biol.*, 55: 635-646.

Befroy, DE (2011). Can Metabolism Be Tracked With MRI Scans? *Disclosures* 21, http://www.medscape.com/viewarticle/751696.

Befroy, DE & Shulman, GI. (2011). Magnetic resonance spectroscopy studies of human metabolism. *Diabetes,* 60: 1361-1369.

Blümler, P; Windt, CW; van Dusschoten D. (2009). Magnetic resonance of plants. *Nova Acta Leopold*, 96: 17-30.

Boer, VO; Luijten, PR; Klomp, DWJ. (2013). Refocused double-quantum editing for lactate detection at 7 T. *Magn. Reson. Med.*, 69: 1-6.

Borisjuk, L; Neuberger, T; Schwender, J; Heinzel, N; Sunderhaus, S; Fuchs, J; Hay, JO; Tschiersch, H; Braun, HP; Denolf, P; Lambert, B; Jakob, PM; Rolletschek, H. (2013). Seed architecture shapes embryo metabolism in oilseed rape. *Plant Cell,* 25: 1625-40.

Borisjuk, L; Rolletschek, H; Neuberger, T. (2013a). Nuclear magnetic resonance imaging of lipid in living plants. *Prog. Lipid Res.*, 52: 465-487.

Borisjuk, L; Rolletschek, H; Neuberger, T. (2012). Surveying the plant's world by magnetic resonance imaging. *Plant J.,* 70:129-46.

Boss, A; Bisdas, S; Kolb, A; Hofmann, M; Ernemann, U; Claussen, CD; Pfannenberg, C; Pichler, BJ; Reimold, M; Stegger, L. (2010). Hybrid PET/MRI of intracranial masses: initial experiences and comparison to PET/CT. *J. Nucl. Med.*, 51: 1198-1205.

Bottomley, AP. (1984a). Selective volume method for performing localized NMR spectroscopy. *US Patent* 1984.

Bottomley, AP; Foster, TH; Leue, WM. (1984b). In vivo nuclear magnetic resonance chemical shift imaging by selective irradiation. *Proc. Natl. Acad. Sci. USA*, 81: 6856-6860.

Brescia, MA; Pugliese, T; Hardy, E; Sacco, A. (2007). Compositional and structural investigations of ripening of table olives, Bella della Daunia, by means of traditional and magnetic resonance imaging analyses. *Food Chemistry*, 105: 400-404.

Bringmann, G; Wolf, K; Meininger, M; Rokitta, M; Haase A. (2001). In vivo 19F NMR chemical-shift imaging of Ancistrocladus species. *Protoplasma,* 218: 134-143.

Brown, TR; Kincaid, BM; Ugurbil, K. (1982). NMR chemical shift imaging in three dimensions. *Proc. Natl. Acad. Sci. USA*, 79: 3523-3526.

Bühler, J; Huber, G; Schmid, F; Blümler P. (2011). Analytical model for long-distance tracer-transport in plants. *J. Theor. Biol.*, 270: 70-79.

Büscher, K; Judenhofer, MS; Kuhlmann, MT; Hermann, S; Wehrl, HF; Schäfers, KP; Schäfers, M; Pichler, BJ; Stegger, L. (2010). Isochronous assessment of cardiac metabolism and function in mice using hybrid PET/MRI. *J. Nucl. Med.*, 51: 1277-1284.

Callaghan, PT. (1991). Principles of nuclear magnetic resonance microscopy (Oxford [England]; New York: Clarendon Press ; Oxford University Press).

Callaghan, PT; Clarke, CJ; Forde, LC. (1994). Use of static and dynamic NMR microscopy to investigate the origins of contrast in images of biological tissues. *Biophys. Chem.*, 50: 225-235.

Cerutti, E; Viale, A; Damont, A; Dollé, F; Aime S. (2011). Synthesis and testing of a p-H2 hyperpolarized 13C probe based on the pyrazolo[1,5-a]pyrimidineacetamide DPA-713, an MRI vector to target the peripheral benzodiazepine receptors. *Magn. Reson. Chem.*, 49: 795-800.

Cha, S; Zhang, H; Ilarslan, HI; Wurtele, ES; Brachova, L; Nikolau, BJ; Yeung, ES. (2008). Direct profiling and imaging of plant metabolites in intact tissues by using colloidal graphite-assisted laser desorption ionization mass spectrometry. *Plant J.,* 55: 348-60.

Chatziioannou, AF. (2002). PET scanners dedicated to molecular imaging of small animal models. *Mol. Imaging Biol.*, 4: 47-63.

Chen, AP; Albers, MJ; Cunningham, CH; Kohler, SJ; Yen, YF; Hurd, RE; Tropp, J; Bok, R; Pauly, JM; Nelson, SJ et al. (2007). Hyperpolarized C-13 spectroscopic imaging of the TRAMP mouse at 3T-initial experience. *Magn. Reson. Med.*, 58: 1099-1106.

Chen, J; Lanza, GM; Wickline SA. (2010). Quantitative magnetic resonance fluorine imaging: today and tomorrow. *Wiley Interdiscip Rev. Nanomed Nanobiotechnol.*, 2: 431-440.

Chudek, JA & Hunter, G. (1997). Magnetic resonance imaging of plants. *Prog Nucl. Magn. Reson. Spectrosc.*, 31: 43-62.

Connelly, A; Lohman, JAB; Loughman, BC; Quiquampoix, H; Ratcliffe, RG. (1987). High resolution imaging of plant tissue by NMR. *J. Exp. Bot.*, 38: 1713-1723.

Cudalbu, C; Comment, A; Kurdzesau, F; van Heeswijk, RB; Uffmann, K; Jannin, S; Denisov, V; Kirik, D; Gruetter, R. (2010). Feasibility of in vivo 15N MRS detection of hyperpolarized 15N labeled choline in rats. *Phys. Chem. Chem. Phys.*, 12: 5818-5823.

Damadian, RV. (1971). Tumor Detection by Nuclear Magnetic Resonance. *Science*, 171: 1151-1153.

Day, SE; Kettunen, MI; Gallagher, FA; Hu, DE; Lerche, M; Wolber, J; Golman, K; Ardenkjaer-Larsen, JH; Brindle KM. (2007). Detecting tumor response to treatment using hyperpolarized 13C magnetic resonance imaging and spectroscopy. *Nat. Med.*, 13: 1382-1387.

De Graaf, RA. (2007). In vivo NMR Spectroscopy. Principles and Techniques, 2nd edn. Chichester: John Wiley & Sons Ldt.

De Graaf, RA; Rothman, DL; Behar, KL. (2011). State of the art direct 13C and indirect 1H-[13C] NMR spectroscopy in vivo. A practical guide. *NMR Biomed.*, 24: 958-972.

De Schepper, V; Bühler, J; Thorpe, M; Roeb, G; Huber, G; van Dusschoten, D; Jahnke, S; Steppe, K. (2013). 11C-PET imaging reveals transport dynamics and sectorial plasticity of oak phloem after girdling. *Front Plant Sci.*, 4: 200.

Dörr, JR; Yu, Y; Milanovic, M; Beuster, G; Zasada, C; Däbritz, JH; Lisec,J; Lenze, D; Gerhardt, A; Schleicher, K; Kratzat, S; Purfürst, B; Walenta, S; Mueller-Klieser, W; Gräler, M; Hummel, M; Keller, U; Buck, AK; Dörken, B; Willmitzer, L; Reimann, M; Kempa, S; Lee, S; Schmitt, CA. (2013). Synthetic lethal metabolic targeting of cellular senescence in cancer therapy. *Nature,* doi:10.1038/nature12437.

Dydak, U; Pruessmann, KP; Weiger, M; Tsao, J; Meier, D; Boesiger, P. (2003). Parallel spectroscopic imaging with spin-echo trains. *Magn. Reson. Med.*, 50: 196-200.

Elliot, I & Skerrit, G. (2006). Handbook of Veterinary MRI (Malden, Mass.: Blackwell Publishing).

Fiorani, F & Schurr, U. (2013). Future Scenarios for Plant Phenotyping. *Annu. Rev. Plant Biol.*, 64: 267-291.

Formica, D & Silvestri, S. (2004). Biological effects of exposure to magnetic resonance imaging: an overview. *Biomed Eng Online*, 3: 11.

Fox, GG; Ratcliffe, RG; Robinson, SA; Slade, AP; Stewart, GR. (1992). Detection of 15N-labeled ammonium. In Vivo, 15N NMR versus mass spectrometry. *J. Magn. Reson.*, 96: 146-153.

Frahm, J; Merboldt, KD; Hänicke, W. (1987). Localized proton spectroscopy using stimulated echoes. *J. Magn. Reson.*, 72: 502-508.

Friis, EM; Crane, PR; Pedersen, KR; Bengtson, S; Donoghue, PCJ; Grimm, GW; Stampanoni, M. (2007). Phase-contrast X-ray microtomography links Cretaceous seeds with Gnetales and Bennettitales. *Nature,* 450: 549-552.

Furuya, Y; Ikehira, H; Obata, T; Koga, M; Yoshida K. (1997). The measurement of blood flow parameters with deuterium stable isotope MR imaging. *Ann. Nucl. Med.*, 11: 281-284.

Fuchs, J, Neuberger, T, Rolletschek, H, Schiebold, S, Nguyen, TH, Borisjuk, N, Börner, A, Melkus, G, Jakob, P, Borisjuk, L. (2013). A non-invasive platform for imaging and quantifying oil storage in submillimetre tobacco seed. *Plant Physiol.*, 161: 583-93.

Gallagher, FA; Kettunen, MI; Day, SE; Hu, D; Karlsson, M; Gisselsson, A; Lerche, MH; Brindle, KM. (2011). Detection of tumor glutamate metabolism in vivo using (13)C magnetic resonance spectroscopy and hyperpolarized [1-(13)C]glutamate. *Magn. Reson. Med.,* 66: 18-23.

Garwood, M & DelaBarre, L. (2001). The return of the frequency sweep: designing adiabatic pulses for contemporary NMR. *J. Magn. Reson.*, 153: 155-177.

Gatehouse, PD & Bydder, GM. (2003). Magnetic resonance imaging of short T2 components in tissue. *Clin. Radiol.*, 58: 1-19.

Gersbach, PV & Reddy, N. (2002). Non-invasive localization of thymol accumulation in Carum copticum (Apiaceae) fruits by chemical shift selective magnetic resonance imaging. *Ann. Bot.*, 90: 253-257.

Gilad, AA; Ziv, K; McMahon, MT; van Zijl, PCM; Neeman, M; Bulte, JWM. (2008). MRI reporter genes. *J. Nucl. Med.*, 49: 1905-1908.

Glidewell, SM; Möller, M; Duncan, G; Mill, RR; Masson, D; Williamson, B. (2002). NMR imaging as a tool for noninvasive taxonomy: comparison of female cones of two Podocarpaceae. *New Phytol.*, 154: 197-207.

Gode, D & Volmer, DA. (2013). Lipid imaging by mass spectrometry – a review. *Analyst,* 138: 1289-315.

Golman, K; Zandt, RI; Thaning, M. (2006a). Real-time metabolic imaging. *Proc. Natl. Acad. Sci. USA*,103: 11270-11275.

Golman, K; Zandt, RI; Lerche, M; Pehrson, R; Ardenkjaer-Larsen, JH. (2006b). Metabolic imaging by hyperpolarized 13C magnetic resonance imaging for in vivo tumor diagnosis. *Cancer Res*, 66: 10855-10860.

Govindaraju, V; Young, K; Maudsley, AA. (2000). Proton NMR chemical shifts and coupling constants for brain metabolites. *NMR Biomed.*, 13: 129-153.

Gussoni, M; Greco, F; Vezzoli, A; Osuga, T; Zetta, L. (2001). Magnetic resonance imaging of molecular transport in living morning glory stems. *Magn. Reson. Imaging*, 19: 1311-1322.

Haacke, EM; Brown, R; Thomson, M; Venkatesan, R. (1999). Magnetic resonance imaging: physical principles and sequence design (New York: John Wiley & Sons LTD).

Haacke, EM & Liang, ZP. (2000). Challenges of imaging structure and function with MRI. *IEEE Eng. Med. Biol. Mag*, 19: 55-62.

Haase, A; Frahm, J; Hänicke, W; Matthaei D. (1985). 1H NMR chemical shift selective (CHESS) imaging. *Phys Med. Biol.*, 30: 341-344.

Halloin, JM; Cooper, TG; Potchen, EJ; Thompson, TE. (1993). Proton magnetic resonance imaging of lipid in pecan embryos. *J. Am. Oil Chem. Soc.*, 70: 1259-62.

Haneder, S; Konstandin, S; Morelli, JN; Nagel, AM; Zoellner, FG; Schad, LR; Schoenberg, SO; Michaely, HJ. (2011). Quantitative and Qualitative 23Na MR Imaging of the Human Kidneys at 3 T: Before and after a Water Load. *Radiology,* 260: 857-865.

Hardy, CJ & Dumoulin CL. (1987). Lipid and water suppression by selective 1H homonuclear polarization transfer. *Magn. Reson. Med.*, 5: 58-66.

Hart, AG; Bowtell, RW; Köckenberger, W; Wenseleers, T; Ratnieks, FL. (2003). Magnetic resonance imaging in entomology: a critical review. *J. Insect Sci.,* 3: 5.

He, Q; Shungu, DC; van Zijl, PC; Bhujwalla, ZM; Glickson, JD. (1995). Single-scan in vivo lactate editing with complete lipid and water suppression by selective multiple-quantum-coherence transfer (Sel-MQC) with application to tumors. *J. Magn. Reson. B,* 106: 203-211.

Heidenreich, M; Köckenberger, W; Kimmich, R; Chandrakumara, N; Bowtell, R. (1998). Investigation of carbohydrate metabolism and transport in castor bean seedlings by cyclic J cross polarization imaging and spectroscopy. *J. Magn. Reson.*, 132: 109-124.

Hinshaw, WS; Bottomley, PA; Holland, GN. (1977). Radiographic thinsection image of the human wrist by nuclear magnetic resonance. *Nature*, 270: 722-723.

Hinshaw, WS; Bottomley, PA; Holland, GN. (1979). A demonstration of the resolution of NMR imaging in biological systems. *Experientia,* 35: 1268-1269.

Hisa, Y; Tatemoto, K; Dejima, K; Nishiyama, Y; Masuda, Y; Ikuta, H. (1994). Magnetic resonance imaging for aspirated peanut in the broncus. *J. Laryngol Otol.,* 108: 804-805.

Hoad, C; Rayment, P; Risse, V; Cox, E; Ciampi, ES; Pregent, L; Marciani, L; Butler, M; Spiller, R; Cowland, P. (2011). Encapsulation of lipid by alginate reduces bio-accessibility: An in vivo 13C breath test and MRI study. *Food Hydrocolloids*, 25: 1190-1200.

Hoad, CL; Marcani, L; Gray, D; Fisk, I; Makkhun, S; Placidi, E; Totman, JJ; Spiller, RC; Cowland, PA. (2008). Non invasive imaging of differing physical forms of dietary fat during digestion in humans. Proc Intl Soc *Mag. Reson. Med.*, 16: 2628.

Horn, PJ, Korte, AR, Neogi, PB, Love, E, Fuchs, J, Strupat, K, Borisjuk, L, Shulaev, V, Lee, YJ, Chapman, KD. (2012). Spatial mapping of lipids at cellular resolution in embryos of cotton. *Plant Cell, 24*: 622-636.

Hu, Q; Noll, RJ; Li, H; Makarov, A; Hardman M; Graham, Cooks R. (2005).The Orbitrap: a new mass spectrometer. *J. Mass Spectrom*, 40: 430-443.

Hu, S; Lustig, M; Chen, AP; Crane, J; Kerr, A; Kelley, DAC; Hurd, R; Kurhanewicz, J; Nelson, SJ; Pauly, JM; Vigneron, DB. (2008). Compressed sensing for resolution enhancement of hyperpolarized 13C flyback 3D-MRSI. *J. Magn. Reson.*, 192: 258-264.

Huang, X; Huang, G; Zhang, S; Sagiyama, K; Togao, O; Ma, X; Wang, Y; Li, Y; Soesbe, TC; Sumer, BD; Takahashi. M; Sherry, AD; Gao J. (2013). Multi-Chromatic pH-Activatable (19) F-MRI Nanoprobes with Binary ON/OFF pH Transitions and Chemical-Shift Barcodes. *Angew Chem. Int. Ed. Engl.,* 52: 8074-8078.

Hugg, JW; Matson, GB; Tweig, DB; Maudsley, AA; Sappey-Marinier, D; Weiner, MW. (1992). 31P MR spectroscopic imaging (MRSI) of normal and pathological human brains. *Magn. Reson. Imag*, 10: 227-243.

Hurd, RE & John, BK. (1991). Gradient-enhanced proton-detected heteronuclear multiple-quantum coherence spectroscopy. *J. Magn. Reson.*, 86: 648-653.

Idiyatullin, D; Corum, C; Moeller, S; Prasad, HS; Garwood, M; Nixdorf DR. (2011). Dental magnetic resonance imaging: making the invisible visible. *J Endod*, 37: 745-752.

Idiyatullin, D; Corum, C; Park, JY; Garwood M. (2006). Fast and quiet MRI using a swept radiofrequency. *J. Magn. Reson.*, 181: 342-349.

Ishida, N; Koizumi, M; Kano, H. (1996). Location of sugars in barley seeds during germination by NMR microscopy. *Plant Cell Environ.*, 19: 1415-1422.

Jahnke, S; Menzel, MI; Van Dusschoten, D; Roeb, GW; Beuhler, J; Minwuyelet, S; Blümler, P; Temperton, VM; Hombach, T; Streun, M ; Beer, S; Khodaverdi, M; Ziemons, K; Coenen, HH; Schurr, U. (2009). Combined MRI-PET dissectsdynamic changes in plant structures and functions. *Plant J.*, 59: 634-644.

Jansen, MA; Van Emous, JG; Nederhoff, MG and Van Echteld, CJ. (2004). Assessment of myocardial viability by intracellular 23Na magnetic resonance imaging. *Circulation,* 110: 3457-3464.

Jenner, CF; Xia, Y; Eccles, CD; Callaghan, PT. (1988). Circulation of water within wheat grain revealed by nuclear magnetic resonance micro-imaging. *Nature*, 336: 399-402.

Jun, JH; Song, Z; Liu, Z; Nikolau, BJ; Yeung, ES; Lee, YJ. (2010). High-spatial and high-mass resolution imaging of surface metabolites of Arabidopsis thaliana by laser desorption–ionization mass spectrometry using colloidal silver. *Anal. Chem.*, 82: 3255-3265.

Kalusche, B; Verscht, J; Gebauer, G; Komor, E; Haase, A. (1999). Sucrose unloading in the hypocotyl of the Ricinus communis L. seedling measured by 13C-nuclear magnetic resonance spectroscopy in vivo. *Planta,* 208: 358-364.

Kampf, T; Fischer, A; Basse-Lüsebrink, TC; Ladewig, G; Breuer, F; Stoll, G; Jakob, PM, Bauer, WR. (2010). Application of compressed sensing to in vivo 3D 19F CSI. *J. Magn. Reson.*, 207: 262-273.

Kanamori, K & Ross, BD. (1997). Glial alkalinization detected in vivo by 1H-15N heteronuclear multiple-quantum coherence-transfer NMR in severely hyperammonemic rat. *J. Neurochem.*, 68: 1209-1220.

Kanamori, K & Ross, BD. (1999). Localized 15N NMR spectroscopy of rat brain by ISIS. *Magn. Reson. Med.*, 41: 456-463.

Keutgen, N; Matsuhashi, S; Mizuniwa, C; Ito, T; Fujimura, T; Ishioka, NS; Watanabe, S; Sekine, T; Uchida, H; Hashimoto, S. (2002). Transfer function analysis of positron-emitting tracer imaging system (PETIS) data. *Appl. Radiat. Isot.*, 57: 225-233.

Khatib-Shahidi, S; Andersson, M; Herman, JL; Gillespie, TA; Caprioli, RM. (2006). Direct molecular analysis of whole-body animal tissue sections by imaging MALDI mass spectrometry. *Anal. Chem.*, 78: 6448-6456.

Kinchesh, P & Ordidge, RJ. (2005). Spin-echo MRS in humans at high field: LASER localisation using FOCI pulses. *J. Magn. Reson.*, 175: 30-43.

Kiser, MR; Reid, CD; Crowell, AS; Phillips, RP; Howell, CR. (2008). Exploring the transport of plant metabolites using positron emitting radiotracers. *HFSP Journal* 2, 4: 189-204.

Kiyomiya, S; Kiyomiya, S; Nakanishi, H; Uchida, H; Tsuji, A; Nishiyama, S; Futatsubashi, M; Tsukada, H; Ishioka, NS; Watanabe, S; Ito, T; Mizuniwa, C; Osa, A; Matsuhashi, S; Hashimoto, S; Sekine, T; Mori, S. (2001). Real time visualization of 13N-translocation in rice under different environmental conditions using positron emitting tracer imaging system. *Plant Physiol.*, 125: 1743-1754.

Klomp DW; van de Bank BL; Raaijmakers A; Korteweg MA; Possanzini C; Boer VO; van de Berg CA; van de Bosch MA; Luijten PR. (2011). 31P

MRSI and 1H MRS at 7 T: initial results in human breast cancer. *NMR Biomed.* 24: 1337-1342.

Köckenberger W & Granwehr J. (2009). MR microscopy. In Encyclopedia of Spectroscopy and Spectrometry (Lindon J, Tranter G and Koppenaal D, eds.). London: Academic Press, pp. 1654-1662.

Köckenberger W. (2001). Functional imaging of plants by magnetic resonance experiments. *Trends Plant Sci*, 6: 286-292.

Köckenberger W; De Panfilis CD; Dahiya P; Rawsthorne S. (2004). High resolution NMR microscopy of plants and fungi. *J. Microsc.*, 214: 182-189.

Kopp, C; Linz, P; Dahlmann, A; Hammon, M; Jantsch, J; Müller, DN; Schmieder, RE; Cavallaro, A; Eckardt, KU; Uder, M; Luft, FC; Titze, J. (2013). 23Na Magnetic Resonance Imaging-Determined Tissue Sodium in Healthy Subjects and Hypertensive Patients. *Hypertension,* 61: 635-640.

Lau, AZ; Chen, AP; Gu, Y; Ladouceur-Wodzak, M.; Nayak, KS; Cunningham, CH. (2013). Noninvasive identification and assessment of functional brown adipose tissue in rodents using hyperpolarized (13)C imaging. *Int J Obes* (Lond), doi: 10.1038/ijo.2013.58.

Lee, YJ; Perdian, DC; Song, Z; Yeung, ES; Nikolau, BJ. (2012). Use of mass spectrometry for imaging metabolites in plants. *Plant J.,* 70: 81-95.

Levitt MH. (2008). Spin dynamics: basics of nuclear magnetic resonance. (Chichester, England; Hoboken, NJ: John Wiley & Sons).

Li, B; Knudsen C; Hansen, NK; Jørgensen, K; Kannangara, R; Bak, S; Takos, A; Rook, F; Hansen, SH; Møller, BL; Janfelt, C; Bjarnholt, N. (2013). Visualizing metabolite distribution and enzymatic conversion in plant tissues by desorption electrospray ionization mass spectrometry imaging. *Plant J.,* 74: 1059-1071.

Link, J & Seelig, J. (1990). Comparison of deuterium NMR imaging methods and application to plants. *J. Magn. Reson.*, 89: 310-330.

Litt, L. (1995). A nuclear magnetic resonance advance. Imaging fluorinated anesthetics in the brain. *Anesthesiology,* 83: 651-653.

Liu, S; Shah, SJ; Wilmes, LJ; Feiner, J; Kodibagkar, VD; Wendland, MF; Mason, RP; Hylton, N; Hopf, HW; Rollins, MD. (2011). Quantitative tissue oxygen measurement in multiple organs using 19F MRI in a rat model. *Magn. Reson. Med.*, 66: 1722-1730.

Lockhart, SH; Cohen, Y; Yasuda, N; Freire, B; Taheri, S; Litt, L, Eger EI 2nd. (1991). Cerebral uptake and elimination of desflurane, isoflurane, and halothane from rabbit brain: an in vivo NMR study. *Anesthesiology,* 74: 575-580.

Louie, KB; Bowen, BP; Alhany, SMc; Huang, Y; Price, JC; Mao, J; Hellerstein, M; Northen, R. (2013). Mass spectrometry imaging for in situ kinetic histochemistry. *Sci. Rep.,* 3: 1656.

Ma, D; Gulani, V; Seiberlich N; Liu, K; Sunshine, JL; Duerk, JL; Griswold, MA. (2013). Magnetic resonance fingerprinting. *Nature*, 495: 187-192.

Mansfeld, P & Pykett, IL. (1978). Biological and medical imaging by NMR. *J. Magn. Reson.*, 29: 355-373.

Mansfield, P & Maudsley, AA. (1977). Medical imaging by NMR. *Br. J. Radiol.,* 50: 188-194.

Masad, IS & Grant, SC. (2011). A retunable surface coil for high field 31P and 1H magnetic resonance evaluations of the living mouse leg. *Physiol. Meas*, 32: 1061-1081.

Mason, RP; Hunjan, S; Constantinescu, A; Song, Y; Zhao, D; Hahn, EW; Antich, PP; Peschke, P. (2003). Tumor oximetry: comparison of 19F MR EPI and electrodes. *Adv. Exp. Med. Biol.*, 530: 19-27.

McDonnell, LA & Heeren, RMA. (2007). Imaging mass spectrometry. Mass Spectrom Rev, 26: 606-643.

McRobbie, DW; Moore, EA; Graves, MJ; Prince, MR. (2006). MRI from picture to proton (2nd edition). Cambridge, UK: Cambridge University Press.

Melkus, G; Mörchel, P; Behr, VC; Kotas, M; Flentje, M; Jakob, PM. (2008). Short echo spectroscopic imaging combined with lactate editing in a single scan. *NMR Biomed.*, 21: 1076-1086.

Melkus, G; Mörchel, P; Behr, VC; Kotas, M; Flentje, M; Jakob, PM. (2009a). Sensitive J-Coupled Metabolite Mapping Using Sel-MQC with Selective Multi Spin Echo Readout. *Magn. Reson. Med.*, 62: 880-887.

Melkus, G; Rolletschek, H; Fuchs, J; Radchuk, V; Grafahrend-Belau, E; Sreenivasulu, N; Rutten, T; Weier, D; Heinzel, N; Schreiber, F; Altmann, T; Jakob, PM; Borisjuk, L. (2011). Dynamic 13C/1 H NMR imaging uncovers sugar allocation in the living seed. *Plant Biotechnol. J.*, 9: 1022-1037.

Melkus, G; Rolletschek, H; Radchuk, R; Fuchs, J; Rutten, T; Wobus, U; Altmann, T; Jakob, P; Borisjuk, L. (2009b). The metabolic role of the legume endosperm: a noninvasive imaging study. *Plant Physiol.*, 151: 1139-1154.

Metzler, A; Izquierdo, M; Ziegler, A; Köckenberger, W; Komor, E; von Kienlin M; Haase, A; Decorps, M. (1995). Plant histochemistry by correlation peak imaging. *Proc. Natl. Acad. Sci. USA,* 92: 11912-11915.

Minchin PEH & Thorpe MR. (2003). Using the short-lived isotope C-11 in mechanistic studies of photosynthate transport. *Funct Plant Bio*, 30: 831-841.

Miura, D; Fujimura, Y; Wariishi, H. (2012). In situ metabolomic mass spectrometry imaging: recent advances and difficulties (animals). *J. Proteomics,* 75: 5052-5060.

Mlynárik, V; Gambarota, G; Frenkel, H, Gruetter R. (2006). Localized short-echo-time proton MR spectroscopy with full signal-intensity acquisition. *Magn. Reson. Med.*, 56: 965-970.

Moon, RB & Richards JH. (1973). Determination of intracellular pH by 31P magnetic resonance. *J. Biol. Chem.*, 248: 7276-7278.

Mullendore, DL; Windt, CW; Van As, H; Knoblauch, M. (2010). Sieve tube geometry in relation to phloem flow. *Plant Cell,* 22: 579-593.

Müller, T; Oradu, S; Demian, R; Ifa, R; Cooks, G; Kräutler, B. (2011). Direct Plant Tissue Analysis and Imprint Imaging by Desorption Electrospray Ionization Mass Spectrometry. *Anal. Chem.*, 83: 5754-5761.

Nakanishi, TM; Okuni, Y; Furukawa, J; Tanoi, K; Yokota, H; Ikeue, N; Matsubayash, M; Uchida, H; Tsiji, A. (2003). Water movement in a plant sample by neutron beam analysis as well as positron emission tracer imaging system. *J. Radioanal Nucl. Chem.*, 255: 149-153.

Nelson, SJ; Kurhanewicz, J; Vigneron, DB; Larson, PEZ; Harzstark, AL; Ferrone, M; van Criekinge, M; Chang, JW, Bok, R, Park, I, Reed, G, Carvajal, L, Small, EJ, Munster, P, Weinberg, VK, Ardenkjaer-Larsen, JH, Chen, AP, Hurd, RE, Odegardstuen, LI, Robb, FJ, Tropp, J, Murray, JA. (2013). Metabolic Imaging of Patients with Prostate Cancer Using Hyperpolarized [1-13C] Pyruvate. *Sci. Transl. Med.*, doi: 10.1126/ scitranslmed.3006070.

Neuberger, T & Webb, AG. (2009b). Radiofrequency coils for magnetic resonance microscopy and microimaging. *NMR Biomed.*, 22: 975-981.

Neuberger, T; Gulani, V, Webb, A. (2007). Sodium renal imaging in mice at high magnetic fields. *Magn. Reson. Med.*, 58: 1067-1071.

Neuberger, T; Rolletschek, H; Webb, A; Borisjuk, L. (2009a). Non-invasive mapping of lipids in plant tissue using magnetic resonance Imaging. In Lipidomics, Methods and Protocols. Edited by Armstrong D. Humana Press: 485-496.

Neuberger, T; Sreenivasulu, N; Rokitta, M; Rolletschek, H; Göbel, C; Rutten, T; Radchuk, V; Feussner, I; Wobus, U; Jakob, P; Webb, A; Borisjuk, L. (2008). Quantitative imaging of oil storage in developing crop seeds. *Plant Biotechnol. J.*, 6: 31-45.

Nimesh, S; Mohottalage, S; Vincent, R; Kumarathasan, P. (2013). Current status and future perspectives of mass spectrometry imaging. *Int. J. Mol. Sci.,* 14: 11277-11301.

Obata, T; Ikehira, H; Koga, M; Yoshida, K; Kimura, F; Tateno, Y. (1995). Deuterium magnetic resonance imaging of rabbit eye in vivo. *Magn. Reson. Med.,* 33: 569-572.

Ohtake, N; Sato, T; Fujikake, H; Sueyoshi, K; Ohyama, T; Ishioka, NS; Watanabe, S; Osa, A; Sekine, T; Matsuhashi, S; Ito, T; Mizuniwa, C; Kume, T; Hashimoto, S; Uchida, H; Tsuji, A. (2001). Rapid N transport to pods and seeds in N-deficient soybean plants. *J. Exp. Bot.*, 52: 277-283.

Olt, S; Krötz, E; Komor, E; Rokitta, M; Haase, A. 23Na and (1)H NMR microimaging of intact plants. (2000). *J. Magn. Reson.*, 144: 297-304.

Ordidge, R; Connelly, A; Lohman, JA. (1986). Image-selected in Vivo spectroscopy (ISIS). A new technique for spatially selective nmr spectroscopy. *J. Magn. Reson.*, 66: 283-294.

Osuga, T & Tatsuoka, H. (1999). Effect of 1.5 T steady magnetic field on neuroconduction of a bullfrog sciatic nerve in a partially active state within several hours after extraction. *Magn. Reson. Imaging*, 17: 791-794.

Patrick, JW & Offler, CE. (2001). Compartmentation of transport and transfer events in developing seeds. *J. Exp. Bot.*, 52: 551-564.

Paul, AL; Ferl, RJ; Meisel, MW. (2006). High magnetic field induced changes of gene expression in arabidopsis. *Bio Magn Res. Technol.*, 4:7.

Phelps ME. (2004). PET: Molecular Imaging and Its Biological Applications. New York: Springer-Verlag, edited by Michael E. Phelps: 621p.

Phelps, ME; Hoffman, EJ; Mullani, NA; Ter-Pogossian, MM. (1975). Application of annihilation coincidence detection to transaxial reconstruction tomography. *J. Nuc. Med.*,16: 210-224.

Pohmann, R; von Kienlin, M; Haase, A. (1997). Theoretical evaluation and comparison of fast chemical shift imaging methods. *J. Magn. Reson.*, 129: 145-160.

Pope, JM; Jonas, D; Walker, RR. (1993). Applications of NMR micro-imaging to the study of water, lipid and carbonhydrate distribution in grape berries. *Protoplasma*, 173: 177-186.

Pope, JM; Rumpel, H; Kuhn, W; Walker, R; Leach, D; Sarafis, V. (1991). Application of chemical-shift-selective NMR microscopy to the non-invasive histochemistry of plant materials. *Magn. Reson. Imaging*, 9: 357-363.

Posse, S; Otazo, R; Dage,r SR; Alger, J. (2013). MR spectroscopic imaging: principles and recent advances. *J. Magn. Reson. Imag*, 37: 1301-1325.

Ratcliffe, RG & Roscher, A. (1998). Prospects for in vivo NMR methods in xenobiotic research in plants. *Biodegradation,* 9: 411-422.

Rautiainen, J; Lehto, LJ; Tiitu, V; Kiekara, O; Pulkkinen, H; Brünott, A; van Weeren, R; Brommer, H; Brama, PA; Ellermann, J; Kiviranta, I; Nieminen, MT; Nissi, MJ. (2013). Osteochondral Repair: Evaluation with Sweep Imaging with Fourier Transform in an Equine Model. *Radiology.* [Epub ahead of print].

Rohren, EM; Turkington, TG; Coleman, RE. (2004). Clinical applications of PET in oncology. *Radiology* 231: 305-332.

Rolletschek, H; Melkus, G; Grafahrend-Belau, E; Fuchs, J; Heinzel, N; Schreiber, F; Jakob, PM; Borisjuk, L. (2011). Combined noninvasive imaging and modeling approaches reveal metabolic compartmentation in the barley endosperm. *Plant Cell,* 23: 3041-3054.

Rothman, DL; Behar, KL; Hetherington, HP; Shulman, RG. (1984). Homonuclear 1H double-resonance difference spectroscopy of the rat brain in vivo. *Proc. Natl. Acad. Sci. USA*, 81: 6330-6334.

Ruiz-Cabello, J; Barnett, BP; Bottomley, PA; Bulte, JW. (2011). Fluorine (19F) MRS and MRI in biomedicine. *NMR Biomed.*, 24: 114-129.

Sacchi, GA; Cocucci, M. (1992). Effects of deuterium oxide on growth, proton extrusion, potassium influx, and in vitro plasma membrane activities in maize root segments. *Plant Physiology*, 100: 1962-1967.

Schaub, TM; Hendrickson, CL; Horning, S; Quinn, JP; Senko, MW; Marshall, AG. (2008). High-performance mass spectrometry: Fourier transform ion cyclotron resonance at 14.5 Tesla. *Anal. Chem.*, 80: 3985-3990.

Schiebold, S; Tschiersch, H; Borisjuk, L; Heinzel, N; Radchuk, R; Rolletschek, H. (2011). A novel procedure for the quantitative analysis of metabolites, storage products and transcripts of laser microdissected seed tissues of Brassica napus. *Plant Methods*, 7: 19.

Schwachtje, J; Minchin, PEH; Jahnke, S; van Dongen, JT; Schittko, U; Baldwin, IT. (2006). SNF1-related kinases allow plants to tolerate herbivory by allocating carbon to roots. *Proc. Natl. Acad. Sci. USA*, 103: 12935-12940.

Shrestha, B; Vertes, A. (2009). In situ metabolic profiling of single cells by laser ablation electrospray ionization mass spectrometry. *Anal. Chem.*, 81: 8265-8271.

Skibbe, U; Christeller, JT; Eccles, CD; Laing, WA; Callaghan, PT. (1995). Phosphorus imaging as a tool for studying the pH metabolism in living insects. *J. Magn. Reson.* B, 68: 393-398.

Smith, MA; Koutcher, JA, Zakian KL. (2008). J-difference lactate editing at 3.0 Tesla in the presence of strong lipids. *J. Magn. Reson. Imag*, 28: 1492,1498.

Smiciklas, M. (2012) The Power of Infographics: Using Pictures to Communicate and Connect with Your Audience Always learning Que Biz-Tech Series, Que Publishing; p. 199.

Sotak, C & Freeman, D. (1988). A Method for Volume-Localized Lactate Editing Using Zero-Quantum Coherence Created in a Stimulated-Echo Pulse Sequence. *J. Magn. Reson.*, 77: 382-388.

Streun, M; Beer, S; Ziemons, K. (2007). PlanTIS: a positron emission tomograph for imaging 11C transport in plants. *IEEE Nuclear Science Symposium Conference Record*, 6: 4110–4112.

Streun, M; Brandenburg, G; Larue, H; Parl, C & Ziemons, K. (2006). The data acquisition system of ClearPET Neuro - a small animal PET scanner. *IEEE Trans Nucl. Sci.*, 53: 700-703.

Szimtenings, M; Olt, S; Haase, A. (2003). Flow encoded NMR spectroscopy for quantification of metabolite flow in intact plants. *J. Magn. Reson.*, 161: 70-76.

Tanoi, K; Hojo, J; Nishioka, M; Nakanishi, TM; Suzuki, K. (2005). New technique to trace 15O water uptake in a living plant with an imaging plate and a BGO detector system. *J. Radioanal Nucl. Chem.*, 263: 547-552.

Terekhov, M; Scholz, A; Schreiber, LM. (2013). Measurement of anesthetic uptake kinetics in the brain using (19)F MRI and cross-correlation analysis after pulsed application. *MAGMA*, [Epub ahead of print].

Terskikh, VV; Feurtado, JA; Ren, C; Abrams, SR; Kermode AR. Water uptake and oil distribution during imbibition of seeds of western white pine (Pinus monticola Dougl. ex D. Don) monitored in vivo using magnetic resonance imaging. *Planta,* 221: 17-27.

Ter-Pergossian, M; Phelps, M; Hoffman, E; Mullani, N. (1975). Apositron-emission transaxial tomograph for nuclear imaging (PETT). *Radiology,* 114: 89-98.

Thomas, MA; Hattori, N; Umeda, M; Sawada, T; Naruse, S. (2003). Evaluation of two-dimensional L-COSY and JPRESS using a 3 T MRI scanner: from phantoms to human brain in vivo. *NMR Biomed.*, 16: 245-251.

Thomas, MA; Yue, K; Binesh, N; Davanzo, P; Kumar, A; Siegel, B; Frye, M; Curran, J; Lufkin, R; Martin, P; Guze, P. (2001). Localized two-dimensional shift correlated MR spectroscopy of human brain. *Magn. Reson. Med.*, 46: 58-67.

Tkác, I; Starcuk, Z; Choi, IY; Gruetter, R. (1999). In vivo 1H NMR spectroscopy of rat brain at 1 ms echo time. *Magn. Reson. Med.*, 41: 649-656.

Togao, O; Tsuji, R; Ohno, Y; Dimitrov, I; Takahashi, M. (2010). Ultrashort echo time (UTE) MRI of the lung: assessment of tissue density in the lung parenchyma. *Magn. Reson. Med.*, 64: 1491-1498.

Touboul, D; Laprévote, O; Brunelle, A. (2011). Micrometric molecular histology of lipids by mass spectrometry imaging. *Curr. Opin. Chem. Biol.,* 15: 725-32.

Tse, TY; Spanswick, RM; Jelinski, LW. (1996). Quantitative evaluation of NMR and MRI methods to measure sucrose concentrations in plants. *Protoplasma*, 194, 54-62.

Van As, H. (2007). Intact plant MRI for the study of cell water relations, membrane permeability, cell-to-cell and long distance water transport. *J. Exp. Bot.*, 58: 743-756.

Van As, H; Scheenen, T; Vergeldt, FJ. (2009). MRI of intact plants. *Photosynth Res*, 102: 213-222.

Van As, H & van Duynhoven, J. (2013). MRI of plants and foods. *J. of Magnetic Resonance* 229: 25-34.

Verboven, P; Herremans, E; Borisjuk, L; Helfen, L; Ho, QT; Tschiersch, H; Fuchs, J; Nicolaï, BM; Rolletschek, H. (2013). Void space inside the developing seed of Brassica napus and the modelling of its function. *New Phytol,* 199: 936-47.

Von Kienlin, M; Ziegler, A; Le Fur, Y; Rubin, C; Dećorps, M; Rémy, C. (2000). 2D-spatial/2D-spectral spectroscopic imaging of intracerebral gliomas in rat brain. *Magn. Reson. Med.*, 43: 211-219.

Waiczies, H; Lepore, S; Drechsler, S; Qadri, F; Purfürst, B; Sydow, K; Dathe, M; Kühne, A; Lindel, T; Hoffmann, W; Pohlmann, A; Niendorf, T; Waiczies, S. (2013). Visualizing brain inflammation with a shingled-leg radio-frequency head probe for 19F/1H MRI. *Sci. Reports*, 3: 1280.

Weibel, S; Basse-Luesebrink, TC; Hess, M; Hofmann, E; Seubert, C; Langbein-Laugwitz, J; Gentschev, I; Sturm, VJF; Ye, Y, Kampf, T; Jakob, PM; Szalay, AA .(2013). Imaging of intratumoral inflammation during oncolytic virotherapy of tumors by 19F-magnetic resonance imaging (MRI). *Plos One*, 8 e: 56317 doi: 10.1371/journal.pone.0056317.

Weiger, M; Pruessmann, KP; Hennel, F. (2011). MRI with zero echo time: hard versus sweep pulse excitation. *Magn. Reson. Med.*, 66: 379-389.

Weiss, K; Melkus, G; Jakob, PM; Faber, C. (2009). Quantitative in vivo 1H spectroscopic imaging of metabolites in the early postnatal mouse brain at 17.6 T. *Magma,* 22: 62-72.

Weissleder, R & Pittet, MJ. (2008). Imaging in the era of molecular oncology. *Nature*, 452: 580–589.

Wiseman, JM; Ifa, DR; Cooks, RG. (2008). Desorption electrospray ionization mass spectrometry: Imaging drugs and metabolites in tissues. *PNAS Proc. Natl. Acad. Sci. USA*, 105: 18088-18089.

Wolf, K; van der Toorn, A; Hartmann, K; Schreiber, L; Schwab, W; Haase, A; Bringmann, G. (2000). Metabolite monitoring in plants with double-quantum filtered chemical shift imaging. *J. Exp. Bot.,* 51: 2109-2117.

Xia, Y & Jelinski, LW. (1995) Imaging Low-Concentration Metabolites in the Presence of a Large Background Signal. *J. Magn. Reson.* B, 107: 1-9.

Yoon, JM; Zhao, L; Shanks, JV. (2013). Metabolic Engineering with Plants for a Sustainable Biobased Economy. *Annu. Rev. Chem. Biomol. Eng.,* 4: 211-237.

Zhang, H; Cha, S; Yeung, ES. (2007). Colloidal Graphite-Assisted Laser Desorption/Ionization MS and MSn of Small Molecules. 2. Direct Profiling and MS Imaging of Small Metabolites from Fruits. *Anal. Chem,* 79: 6575-6584.

Ziegler, A; Metzler, A; Köckenberger, W; Izquirdo, M; Komor, E; Haase, A; Decorps, M; von Kienlin, M.(1996). Correlation peak imaging. *J. Magn. Reson. B,* 112: 141-150.

In: *In Vivo* Imaging: New Research
Editors: R. Hough and J. Camarillo
ISBN: 978-1-62948-633-8

Chapter 2

Magnetic-Based Theranostic Nanoparticles: From Hype to Hope

Pericles Pericleous[1], Efstathios P. Efstathopoulos[2], Nikolaos L. Kelekis[2] and Maria Gazouli[3*]
[1]First Department of Surgery,
"Tzaneion" General Hospital, Piraeus, Greece
[2]Second Department of Radiology, School of Medicine,
University of Athens, Greece
[3]Department of Basic Medical Sciences, Laboratory of Biology,
School of Medicine, University of Athens, Athens, Greece

Abstract

The publicity of recently introduced nanoparticles is accelerating in the constantly developing field of cancer research; nanotechnology is being increasingly utilized for the development of breakthrough approaches in terms of cancer diagnosis and therapy. Magnetic nanoparticles offer unprecedented prospect for magnetic separation, nanoparticle-enhanced hyperthermia, targeted drug delivery, regenerative medicine and stem cell therapy and as contrast agents. Magnetic

* Correspondence to: Maria Gazouli, PhD, Michalakopoulou 176, 11527, Athens, Greece, Tel/Fax: +302107462231, e-mail: mgazouli@med.uoa.gr.

resonance imaging (MRI) is an important medical imaging tool, which has the ability to incorporate such contrast agents and provide enhanced clinical information with high spatial and temporal resolutions. Due to its nonionizing radiation, high sensitivity to the distribution of water and other biomolecules and the orientation of fine tissue structures, MRI has been widely applied in clinical practice. Given the recent progress in nanosynthesis and bioengineering, magnetic nanoparticles are expected to serve as an innovative platform, which will enable novel approaches to targeted tumor imaging and therapy. Not only the fabrication of nanoparticles that combine multimodality methods will discard many inadequacies that are present in single-modality imaging methods but also the incorporation of cancer-specific therapeutic payloads will equip these nanoparticles with the ability to provide magnetic-field dependent drug delivery. It is however imperative that, prior to the application of mangetic-based theranostic nanoparticle systems in clinical settings, several key issues need to be addressed, including toxicity, long-term stability and distribution. The aim of this review is to present the latest developments in the design and application of mangetic-based theranostic nanoparticle systems, investigate on their potentially harmful events and explore their future role in personalized medicine.

Keywords: Magnetic nanoperticles, magnetic targeting, targeting agents, magnetic resonance imaging, imaging agents, hyperthermia, therapeutic agents, theranostics

Introduction

The utilization of magnetic nanoparticles in biomedical applications such as magnetic resonance imaging, drug delivery, hyperthermia, tissue engineering and repair, biosensing, biochemical separations and bioanalysis has been thoroughly investigated in recent years. Considerable efforts have been made for their development and understanding of their behaviour while precise control over their synthesis has been applied in order to ensure stability and biocompatibility.

The development of agents which will facilitate simultaneous drug delivery and imaging, commonly known as theranostics, represents an important breakthrough of MNP technology. This review will summarise the latest developments in the design and application of mangetic-based theranostic nanoparticle systems, investigate on their potentially harmful events and explore their future role in personalized medicine.

Design of Magnetic Colloids

There are three main pathways in which magnetic nanoparticles can be synthetised: physical methods (consisting of gas-phase deposisiton and electron beam lithography) [1-4], microbial methods (in which bacteria such as Thermoanaerobacter species and Shewanella species can synthetise Fe3O4 nanoparticles under anaerobic conditions) [5-7] and wet chemical preparation methods (sol-gel method [8, 9], oxidation method [10, 11], chemical coprecipitation [12, 13], hydrothermal method [14, 15], flow injection method [16], electrochemical method [17, 18], aerosol/vapor-phase method [19, 20], sonochemical decomposistion method [21, 22], supercritical fluid method [23, 24] and synthesis using nanoreactors [25, 26]). Lately, metal-doped iron oxides with enhanced magnetic properties have attracted the interest of investigators and various methods have been used for their synthesis [27-19]. Through these systems a broader spectrum of functionalities can be achieved [30-31].

When iron is thinly divided, it becomes extremely reactive towards oxidizing agents and in presence of water and humid air. In order to obtain physically and chemically stable colloidal systems, magnetic nanoparticles have to be protected, usually by means of a surface coating. Coating does not only prevent exposure of MNPs to environmental conditions but also improves their colloidal and physical stability, increases their water-dispersibility and provides functionalisation for further conjugation with targeting ligands or bioactive molecules as well as the ability to construct multifunctional agents [32-36]. The type of the surface coating and its geometric arrangement onto the magnetic core determine the size of the colloid and affect its pharmacokinetics and biodistribution. Surface stabilizing is commonly achieved with the use of nonpolymeric stabilisers based on organic monomers bearing functional groups such as carboxylate, phosphate or sulfate [37-47]. Polymeric coatings have the ability to tailor surface properties of the MNPs (such as chemical functionality and charge) and constitute a barrier to prevent aggregation, thus leading to physically and chemically stable magnetic nanoformulations [48]. PEG is by far the most widely used polymer for nanoparticle coating in nanomedicine due to its nontoxic and impressive steric repulsive properties [49-51]. Apart from PEG, the polysaccharide dextran has also been extensively used for the design of surface coatings of MNPs used in imaging applications in vivo [52-54]. Inorganing metals are also useful for coating. For example, gold-coated IONPs are generally stable under acidic and neutral pH in aqueous media [55]. Moreover, coatings with nonmetallic materials such as graphite have also improved the solubility and stability against oxidation of FeCo colloids in aqueous media [56]. Other coatings consist of SiO2 [57-60], crystalline shells of Fe_3O_4 [61], inorganic matrices such as hydrotalcite or zeolite [62-66]. It is important that key characteristics of coatings must be taken into consideration prior to their use in biomedical applications.

Shell stabilization can also be achieved by generating polymeric shells which are able to avoid cluster growth after nucleation and hold the particle domains apart against attractive forces. The polymeric shell provides functional groups (terminal amine and carboxyl moieties) at the nanoparticle surface allowing further conjugation with bioactive molecules and targeting ligands, thus creating multifunctional MNPs [67-101]. PS/Fe3O4 core/shell nanoparticles of small size and narrow size distribution have been obtained by the polymerization of styrene at the surface of NPs [102], while in situ fabrication of MNPs in the presence of gelatin resulted in the formation of ferrosponges [103]. Hybrid mangetic carriers consisting of alginate SiO2 nanocomposite shell loaded with Fe_3O_4 NPs were found to exhibit superparamagnetic behaviour [104]. Copolymers have also been employed in shell design [105]. Even though these nanoparticles show great potential for drug delivery purposes, caution should be applied during the selection of their materials because the presence of polymers or copolymers during magnetic nanocrystal nucleation and growth may induce imperfections in the crystal structure leading to alteration of magnetic properties of the NPs [106-108].

Liposomes have also been used for the stabilisation of MNPs. Formulation of lipid-like coatings around the magnetic core (mangetoliposomes) can be achieved by taking advantage of the usual liposomal methodologies without any chemical modification of the encapsulated Fe3O4 colloid [109, 110]. Magnetoliposomes can also be obtained from magnetotactic bacteria (bacterial magnetosomes) [111-113]. These MNPs can be utilised in various biomedical applications such as MRI, targeted drug and gene delivery, hyperthermia, magnetic cell separation and development of virus-like particles with high magnetic susceptibility [114-116].

Physicochemical Properties

Geometry plays a pivotal role in the stability of MNPs, both in vivo and in vitro. Size influences the magnetic moment and subsequent response of particles to magnetic fields; a decrease of size results in an increase of the surface area, thus implicating the noncrystaline character of the particles and their magnetic moment [117]. MNPs of very low sizes can exhibit superparamagnetism, which determines greater magnetisation capabilities compared to paramagnetic materials. Size has also been described to control the signal in MRI of iron oxides, affecting the quality of the diagnosis [118, 119]. Apart from geometry, the structure of nanoparticles further defines their magnetic properties and various techniques have been used for its investigation [120-126]

Ferromagnetic particles are those whose unpaired electrons spins align themselves spontaneously in order to exhibit magnetisation without being in a magnetic field. These ferromagnetic materials exhibit permanent magnetisation after they have been removed from a magnetic field. On the contrary, paramagnetic materials are those in which no permanent magnetisation remains once they are removed from a magnetic field. However, ferromagnetic materials exhibit superparamagnetism when they are reduced to particle dimensions smaller than a particular domain. The magnetisation of SPIONs is similar to that of ferromagnetic materials and greater of the one in paramagnetic particles. Thus, superparamagnetic nanomaterials can be easily tracked in a magnetic field without losing the advantage of a stable colloidal suspension [127]. Upon suppresion of the magnetic field, remnant magnetisation of these nanoparticles is greatly reduced or disappears completely and agglomeration can be avoided. Additional benefits of SPIONs result from their heating behaviour when they are exposed to an alternating magnetic field [128] as well as from their powerful enhancement of the proton relaxation times T1 and T2 [129]. On the downside, their reduced size can alter their magnetic properties [130].

Colloidal stability in adequate media is an essential feature for medical applications of MNPs. Because of their moderate average density, MNPs exhibit negligible gravitational settling in the blood flow and in the absence of an applied magnetic field their stability mainly depends on the balance between the act of attractive and repulsive forces [131-134]. Both of these forces could be controlled by engineering of the NPs. When presented in blood, MNPs are exposed to a slightly basic pH and a relatively high ionic strength and these conditions along with the magnetic attractive forces typically lead to particle aggregation. These phenomena can be compensated by electrostatic repulsion between adequately charged surfaces, hydrophilic particle-particle interactions and the existence of an adequate shell onto the particle surface, thus providing in vivo and in vitro stability [135]. When sufficient amount of stabilizing agent is located onto the particle surface, steric stabilization provides adequate stability even at higher electrolyte concentrations and in a wide range of pH values [136].

Pharmacokinetics and Biodistribution

Following IV administration, MNPs used for targeted drug delivery are magnetically guided to the targeted tissue where they remain in situ until the drug is released, while later they undergo clearance from the body. Their transport through the blood vessels is facilitated by the hydrodynamic forces of circulation. Shortly after MNPs enter the circulation, an immediate interaction occurs between them and the plasma proteins which results in the absorption of proteins onto the magnetic colloids (opsonization). This absorption process determines the biological fate of MNPs [137]. The opsonized NPs are captured by macrophages of the liver, spleen and bone marrow (tissues of the reticuloendothelial system) and undergo rapid clearance from the vascular compartment [138-140]. Even though such accumulation favors the instances in which these organs are actually targeted, it is important that rapid clearance should be minimised when nanoparticles need to reach tissues other than those of the RES. This could be achieved via coating [141-142]. PEG is considered to be the most appropriate hydrophilic polymer to date and is commonly used to prevent rapid systemic clearance of NPs [143-145]. It should be noted that, even though early preclinical reports showed no impact on the pharmacokinetic profile of PEGylated lipsosomes after repeated injections [146-147], recent studies document a phenomenon of accelerated blood clearance following repeated injections in rats [148-149]. The ABC phenomenon appears to be dependent on the injected lipid dose (limited or none on high lipid dose) and PEG surface density (no effect at high density) [150]. Additionally, the phenomenon was also reported for PEGylated PLA NPs but was not observed with doxorubicin-encapsulated PEGylated liposomes and hydrophilic polymers such as PVP (conjugated to PLA) [151-153].

Long circulating NPs can reach tumour sites by passive extravasation by taking advantage of the increased tumour permeability which results from the leaky tumour vasculature (Enhanced Permeability and Retention effect) [154-155]. Magnetic force actively guiding MNPs into targeted tumour tissues must be higher than the hydrodynamic blood flow for NPs to avoid rapid clearance [156]. The efficacy of MNP immobilisation also depends on particle size [157].

The importance of size in biodistribution of the intravenously injected MNPs should be taken into consideration during their development. The absorption of opsonins onto the NPs surface and thus their recognition by macrophages and systemic clearance, relates to their size. It had been shown that the systemic clearance of the smaller NPs was slower than that of the bigger NPs [158]. Moreover, NPs above 200nm undergo filtration in the spleen whereas those below 50-100nm will more probably be trapped in the liver [159-164]. Particles with a diameter that exceeds 4μm are mainly captured in the lungs and pose the risk of pulmonary embolism [165].

Surface charge plays and important role in their biodistribution after they enter circulation. Neutral charge interacts minimally with the plasma proteins and prolongs circulation time. On the contrary, a high surface charge (either positive or negative) enhances phagocytic processes [166]. A study carried out on mice showed that strong negative surface charges increased their hepatic uptake [162] whereas positive charges led to particles nonspecifically been attached to cells. Liver uptake has been found to be lower for the electrically neutral particles [167-168].

The administration route may also influence the systemic behaviour of IONPs. When injected locally, small magnetic particles undergo passive infiltration into the interstitial spaces and are gradually absorbed by the lymphatic system, making them ideal candidates for lymphatic targeting. PVP-stabilised and fluorescent tagged MNPs administered via inhalation to mice accumulated considerably in the liver, followed by testis, spleen, lung and brain, thus proving that their ability to cross thight blood barriers [169]. Intraperitoneally injected SiO2 coated MNPs were found distributed at high concentration into liver and spleen, followed by kidneys, heart, testes and uterus and in remarkably smaller concentrations in the lungs. Moreover, they were able to pass the blood-brain barrier and accumulate in the brain [170].

Regarding tissue diffusion of MNPs, an average diameter larger than 10nm usually impedes their diffusion through the small vascular pores of healthy endothelium whereas in compromised endothelium (due to artificial means or specific pathologic conditions) NPs with a diameter up to 700nm could penetrate freely [171]. In nanoparticles of similar sizes, it has been shown that the coating material can also influence tissue uptake. Also, the extent of particle uptake may affect the rate of clearance [172-174]. At the cellular level, larger NPs are only captured by cells capable of phagocytosis whereas smaller NPs could have cellular access through pinocytosis [175]. After they enter the cells, IONPs are clustered with lysosomes and degraded into iron and oxygen under the influence of low pH and hydrolytic enzymes. Fe ions from IONPs can be reused by cells via physiological pathways [176].

Toxicity

The toxicity of MNPs could result from various factors which includes their dose, composition, size, structure, solubility, surface chemistry, route of administration, biodegradability, pharmacokinetics and biodistribution. The biocompatibility of a drug nanocarrier is linked not only to the response of the body's immune system but also to the intrinsic toxicity of it and its metabolites. It is important that colloids and their degradation products undergo rapid clearance after drug release has occurred.

The influence of PEG surface coatings was analysed in an *in vitro* study and results showed that uncoated IONPs caused a significant decrease in cell adhesion compared to that of the control cells, whereas PEG-coated NPs did not cause notable change. The uncoated NP-incubated cells exhibited vacuoles in the cytoplasm with disorganised cytoskeleton, membrane abnormalities and disruption. In another study, incubation of dextran coated IONPs caused cytotoxicity and apoptosis similar to that of the uncoated NPs. On the contrary, albumin coated IONPs did not reduce cell viability and exhibited considerably lower toxicity compared to uncoated and dextran coated NPS [177]. However, it has recently been demonstrated that the same coating may have different toxicological implications when applied onto different cores [178], due to the contribution of other parameters, such as size.

The particle size can have different effects on cells in vitro; IONPs with a size of 30nm were shown to exhibit higher toxic effects when compared to the ones with a size of 0.5μm. Additionally, cell damage can be dose-dependent. Higher size NPs showed no toxic effects at lower doses whereas NPs of lower size showed increased mitochondrial damage with subsequent cell death induced by apoptosis in higher doses [179]. Additionally, interactions of uncoated NPs (often negatively charged) with the cell culture medium can result in alterations in the ionic concentration and protein function and may cause cell detachment and cell death [180]. The surface charge of IONPs can influence cell morphology and function. Research has shown that coating of NPs with DMSA (anionic coating) enhanced endocytosis vy various cell types and caused a concentration-dependent decrease in cell adhesion as well as reduction in the viability of the PC12 pheochromocytoma clinal cell line [181].

However, cytotoxicity of anionic IONPs was observed to depend on the nature of surface coating [182].

It should be noted at this point that even though in vitro toxicity observations provide useful information regarding the safety of the NPs, they do not represent in vivo conditions. As a matter of fact, the cytotoxicity can be more pronounced in vitro due to conditions that cause prolonged exposure of cells to NPs and their degradation products. In vivo, biodegradable NPs are continuously eliminated from circulation.

IONPs that enter circulation are uptaken by macrophages residing in RES organs [183] via receptor-mediated endocytosis and are metabolised in lysosomes [184]. The released free iron is then incorporated into iron stores of the body, then gradually found as haemoglobin and in part bound to transferrin and is mostly eliminated slowly via the faecal route [185]. As a consequence, the injection of high amounts of iron may lead to an increased concentration in plasma as a result of the surpassed transferrin iron binding capacity, leading to oxidative stress as well as cardiac and liver toxicity [186].

IONPs stabilised with different coatings have been evaluated for safety following iv administration [187]. The MNPs showed a satisfactory safety profile in different animal species but depending on the dose administered. For examle, Femuroxtran-10 at a dose of 2.6 mg Fe/kg was safe in rats with no changes in haemodynamic parameters whereas 13 mh Fe/kg dose caused slight increase in aortic blood flow but no arrythmia, no disturbance in electrocardiogram and no respiratory toxicity [161]. Treatment related clinical signs were observed only in single, much higher doses whereas repeated smaller doses caused only moderate changes in haematological parameters. In dogs, dose of 200 mg Fe/kg of Ferumoxtran-10 (a dose 75 times higher than that used in MRI in humans) caused slight cardiovascular toxicity, decrease in blood pressure, increase in respiratory rate, increase of cardiac output and moderate increase in urine output and urinary sodium excretion. After injection, the serum iron was increased in rat, monkey and dog but resolved to normal levels after treatment was withdrawn. Toxicological events were similar to all animals. In human cancer patients, iv injected IONPs (100nm sized particles coated with anhydroglucose polymer) were found to be well tolerated. These NPS were loaded with doxorubicin (anticancer drug).

A transient elevation of the serum iron levels was observed but without any toxic symptoms, while the urine iron concentrations were found to be in normal range. A slight skin discoloration was observed but without any other toxicological event due to the application of a magnetic field on the skin surface [188, 189]. Similarly, Ferucabotran after iv injection was found to be safe, except a slight decrease in clotting factor XI activity [190-193]. In another study, minor CNS related side effects were observed [194]. Surface charge affected the interaction between NPs and biological systems. Neutral and negative charged NPs showed lower interaction with plasma proteins whereas positively charged NPs undergo rapid clearance, leading to nonspecific tissue uptake [195-196]. Following intraperitoneal [197] and subcutaneous administration [198], toxicological effects of NPs were found to be dose and coating/charge dependent. Overall, even though IONPs may be considered to be biocompatible, their safety varies according to their physicochemical properties and route of administration and depends extensively on the dose range and frequency.

Drug Delivery

Conventional drug delivery suffers from poor specificity and reduced diffusion through biological barriers thus leading to suboptimal pharmacological activity and high incidence of adverse reactions [199]. On the other hand, drug encapsulation into nanocarriers that are able to circumvent macrophage-rich organs results to prolonged circulation and possible specific translocation into diseased inflammatory tissues [200-201]. Stimuli sensitive carriers allow selective drug delivery to cells, organs and tissues. These colloidal systems are engineered to be able to change their physical properties under exposure to an external stimulus (temperature, pH, ionic strength, magnetic gradient) leading to the enhancement of drug accumulation at the site of delivery. MNPs due to their magnetic field responsiveness and heat generation properties are prime candidates for such drug delivery [202-210]. In general, NPs smaller than 100nm are more suitable for heat-generating purposes because they exhibit better permeability properties while larger particles can be utilised for magnetic targeting, due to their higher sensitivity to magnetic guidance [211].

The drug loading into MNPs is usually carried out by dissolving the drug in either an organic phase in which the shell material is dissolved or in the aqueous phase containing the MNPs [212]. Because the drug payload and the drug-release rate are essential parameters, special attention has to be paid in preparation procedures. The selection of the shell matrix must take into consideration the physicochemical properties of the drug and it needs to allow retention of the drug until it reaches its target as well as further release at the target size. The efficacy of magnetic guidance may depend on the ability to minimize rapid clearance and efficiently cross biological barriers. MNPs should possess sufficient magnetic susceptibility and the force field must be strong enough to ensure transport to the target site. When the drug reaches the site of action, release can occur by simple diffusion from the matrix or through other parameters (enzymatic degradation, pH, temperature etc.) [213-214]. The location of the magnet and the physiology of the host can affect the therapeutic efficacy when an external magnetic field is used for drug delivery purposes [215-217]. The use of implanted magnets is a promising strategy that could optimize delivery of MNPs to selected areas [218-220].

IONPs coated with polymeric, lipidic or inorganic shells were used as drug-delivery carriers for systemic administration of anticancer agents. Superparamagnetic Fe3O4/PCL core/shell NPs containing gemcitabine showed significant antitumor activity in a dose much lower than of free Gem [221]. Similarly, epirubicin coated MNPs, have been successfully used for the treatment of mice with subcutaneusly implanted colon carcinoma or hypernephroma [222]. In another study, following iv administration and in the absence of extracorpeal magnetic field, Dox-loaded thermally cross-linked SPIONs underwent already significant extravasation into tumour sites and less accumulation than free drug into nontarget organs such as liver. The NP formulation was found to be nontoxic whereas the therapetic active dose of free Doc induced liver impairment, lymphatic damage and reduced WBC count [223]. Magnetic liposomes have also been used for a combination of drug delivery and imaging purposes [224-226]. Liposomes exhibit excellent biocompatibility, ability to incorporate both hydrophilic and hydrophobic compounds, stability and ease of surface functionalisation to achieve prolonged circulation and molecular targeting activities [227]. Moreover, magnetic liposomes have been used for efficient liver targeting even when the RES was inhibited, indicating that liver accumulation was due to the external magnetic field rather than unspecific macrophage uptake [228]. In a clinical studiy MNPs of 100nm in diameter loaded with epirubicin were tested in cancer patients, showing increased accumulation of the NPs into the tumors as observed by MRI [229].

When the accumulation of NPs occurs into the organ or tissue due to their physicochemical characteristics targeting is specified as passive whereas in the case of active targeting, the NPs are enabled to accumulate in the intended organ, tissue or cells by using either stimuli-responsive or surface-functionalized nanodevices with homing moieties [230-232]. Peptides [233], proteins [234] and aptamers [235-239] have been employed for tissue-specific targeting. Monoclonal antibodies have also been used to deliver MNPs, despite their larger size, inherent immunogenicity and poor diffusion through body barriers [240-246].

Nanotheranostics are those nanodevices which possess both therapeutic and diagnostic features. After their iv administration, they should be able to deliver the chemotherapeutic agent towards the targeted site while simultaneously allowing monitoring of the response to treatment [247]. The development of magnetic [248-251] and nonmagnetic [252-253] theranostic systems has been documented in recent studies. However, most reports have verified proof-of-concept only in vitro cell cultures rather than in vivo. NPs loaded with a fluorescent agent and the anticancer drug paclitaxel have been used for drug delivery and simultaneous dual optical and MRI applications. Also reported was the design of multifunctional mesoporous SiO2 NPs exhibiting both fluoresence and MRI imaging capabilities. Dox was covalently loaded to the SiO2 overcoat while the fluorescent dye was covalently linked to the shell. Proof of concept was verified in vitro using MCF-7 breast tumor cell line [254]. In an example of in vivo approach, PEGylated PLGA-coated MNPs functionalised with herceptin and loaded with Dox have demonstrated their ability to address the drug to the cancer tissue in vivo with simultaneous MRI [255, 256]. NPs showed an improved antitumor activity compared to controls [257]. Similarly, fumagillin-loaded MNPs surface-functionalised with RGD for in vivo targeting of integrins in MDS-MB-435 tumours were used for simultaneous drug delivery to tumour angiogenesis and imaging [258]. The magnetic core was used only as a contrast agent for MRI, thus no external magnetic field was applied. In another experiment [221], MNPs coated with a PCL shell and loaded with Gem, the tumour targeting was obtained in vivo by employing an extracorpeal magnetic field. MNPs showed similar antitumour efficacy to that of free Gem but with a remarkably lower dose. Recently, a novel platform was developed [251], in which the theranostic particles were constructed by coating IONPs with a lipidic prodrug. These nanoparticles exhibited an impressive anticancer activity with very low doses of anticancer drug after they were intravenously inserted in mice and guided to the target site with the use of an extracorpeal magnetic field. Because of the embedded IONPs, the tumour collapse could be easily visualised by MRI. This promising platform provides the benefits of very high drug loading and sustained release linked to the prodrug nature of the agent as well as ability to magnetically address the drug to the tumour site even without the presence of a homing device.

In pre-clinical studies, locoregional administration of MNPs close to the tumour sites has been shown to efficiently treat VX-2 squamous cell carcinoma in rabbits [259], orthotopic glioma in mice [260] and Yoshida sarcoma in rat tail [261]. The advantage of this approach is that the locoregional injection limits the biodistribution of the NPs and facilitates rapid access to the tumour site in the direction of the blood flow. BMs have also been used for the delivery of therapeutic substances through locoregional administration. These magnerosomes due to their nanosize and paramagnetic properties [262-264] have been utilised as carriers for drugs and DNA [256, 266]. In a different study, a magnetic liposomal formulation was administered to mice orally with the intestine exposed to an external magnetic field. As a result, there was an increased retention of the formulation in the intestine, followed by oral absorption and liver accumulation, when compared to the oral administration in the absence of the magnetic field [267].

MNPs encapsulated into stimuli-sensitive polymeric shells have been proposed as stimuli sensitive drug delivery systems. A Dox loaded MNP formulation exhibiting drug release in response to temperature and pH alterations facilitated an on-off trigger drug release mechanism. When the temperature was below a lower critical solution point, the drug release was slow whereas in greater temperatures the release was biphasic with an initial burst followed by a sustained release. Such behaviour potentially protects the NP formulation from unwanted drug release as long as it is in the systemic compartment, allowing it to reach the tumour site where with the supply of mild heat the polymer matrix becomes prone to degradation and drug is released [268]. In a subsequent report the dextran moiety of the polymer was replaced by chitosan in order to overcome the potential impact of the high solubility of dextran on the drug release [269].

In other applications, MNPs have been loaded with chemotherapeutic agents that either promoted embolization of tumour arteries (inducing hypoxia) [270] or thrombolysis in artificially implanted thrombuses [271] in the arteries of rats. Both of the above studies reported succesful results. IV injected MNP formulations have also resulted in appreciable clot degradation following iv injection of streptokinase-loaded MNPs in a dog, upon exposure to a magnetic field [272]. Furthermore, magnetic nanoparticles loaded with diclofenac sodium have been used for drug delivery to the articular joints [273] whereas a different type of MNPs loaded with proteins and antioxidant enzymes was used against oxidative stress-mediated diseases (i.e., cardiovascular diseases) [274-275]. Finally, an interesting approach in the area of magnetic drug delivery is the introduction of a magnetizable implant into a desired site of the body which will be able to attract magnetic particles following their iv administration thus providing a localised drug effect, minimizing systemic distribution and adverse effects [276]. This approach has been employed recently for coronary re-stenosis drug delivery [277-280]. MNPs directed towards magnetized stents placed in the restenosis affected arteries significantly inhibited the restenosis compared to the control-treated rats in the absence of magnetic field [281].

Radioimmunotherapy involves low doses of radioactive isotopes conjugated to MAb's for cancer treatment. Magnetic engineering of radioimmunoparticles has shown some promise in preclinical studies by improving the tumour delivery of radioimmunoconjugates and by enhancing their therapeutic efficacy [282, 283] MNPs have also served as a tool for combined radioimmunoconjugate delivery and thermal ablation of the neoplastic tissue [284]. Photodynamic therapy is an emerging treatment of solid tumours which involves administration of a light-activatable nontoxic drug (photosynthetizer) followed by laser illumination of the tumour [285]. The photosynthetizer can cause necrosis and tumour cell death via generation of ROS and free radicals by transferring its excitation energy to surrounding oxygen atoms [286, 287]. In order to overcome intrinsic limitations of conventional photodynamic therapy, such as poor solubility of photosynthetizers and insufficient specificity to the tumour site, IOPNs guided by an external field have been employed. For instance, IONPs loaded into a phospholipid emulsion have been used for the delivery of photosynthetizers to a skin cancer [288]. IONPs were also used for guiding the photosynthetizer to the tumour and for simultaneous MRI [289]. Recently Fe3O4/SiO2 core/shell NPs functionalised with phosphorescent iridium complexes have been designed as a new tool for photodynamic therapy. The nanocomposite was versatile in fascilitating MRI, enhancing the spin-orbit coupling in the Ir complex, thereby making it suitable for phosphorescent labeling and simultaneous generation of oxygen singlets for provoking apoptosis of tumour cells [290].

Magnetic fluid hyperthermia involves the injection of a magnetic fluid into a tissue with its subsequent exposure to an alternating magnetic field, allowing heat generation. Heat is generated due to magnetic hysteresis loss, when MNPs are subjected to an AMF of low moderate frequency. Nanoparticles accumulated in tumours could potentially warm up to a temperature that depends on their magnetic properties, on the strength of the magnetic field, on the frequency of oscillation and on the cooling capacity of the blood flow in the tumour [291-295]. The heat released will be diffused to the adjacent tissues as a result of the oscillation of the magnetic moment inside the NPs exposed to the magnetic field. Tumour cells heated at temperatures of

42-45 Celcius are irreversably damaged [296-299] while local heating of a tumour for approximately 30 minutes has been proven sufficient to destroy the tumour tissue [300]. If the temperature exceeds 56 Celcious, it results in thermoablation [301]. The promise of hyperthermia as a minimally invasive treatment of brain tumours has been demonstrated on a glioblastoma rat model [302]. Aminosilane-coated NPs used in the study maintained high temperature and resulted in significant anticancer activity. The survival of treated rats was increased nearly 5 times compared to the untreated control group.

MNPs encapsulated into cationic liposomes have also been used for induction of magnetic fluid hyperthermia. The introduction of MCLs into MM46 mammary tumor-bearing mice with subsequent exposure to AMF cause an increase in temperature up to 45 Celcius at the surface of the tumour, resulting in tumour regression while the tumour response remained improved after repeated cycles. It was also observed that the repeated hyperthermia treatment had also generated anti-tumour immunity because animals resisted the tumour challenge consisting of successive subcutaneous inoculation of the tumour cells [292]. In another experiment of human hepatocellular carcinoma xenograft, the MFH treatment significantly inhibited the tumour proliferation and induced apoptosis [303]. MFH has also been used in combination with chemotherapy in order to further improve the efficiency of anti-tumour response [304-305]. Combination of MFH with external beam radiation therapy has been proposed due to the complementary mechanism of causing cell death following the two treatments [306]. The use of higher temperatures (up to 70 Celcius) following exposure to AMF of higher amplitude results in thermal ablation of the exposed tissues with tumor necrosis and intensive cell destruction [307]. However, caution should be taken in using this approach because the ablation may cause considerable damage to the skin and to the adjacent healthy tissues due to the possible migration of NPs. However, MFH has been proven more effective than radiofrequency ablation by dielectric heating [308]. In addition to the above applications, MHF could also be utilised to enhance the accumulation of anticancer compounds at the neoplastic target area by altering the local tissue permeability [309-313]. The modified microenvironment of the tumour become more accessible to drugs, drug delivery systems or macromolecules [314-316].

In a clinical study, aminosaline-coated IONPs and MFH was used for the treatment of patients suffering from locally recurrent prostate cancer [316]. Clinicall studies that followed examined the safety of MFH treatment and the quality of life of the patients [317, 318]. Overall, the treatment was found to be well tollerated with a noted moderate treatment-related morbidity and temporary impairment of quality of life due to urinary problems and tiredness. It should also be noted that symptoms resolved a few weeks after therapy. In a different clinical trial, MFH was carried out on patients with various neoplastic diseases by using a whole-body magnetic field applicator and magnetic fluid composed of aminosaline-coated IONPs [319] and, finally, MFH was also experienced on patients with miltiforme glioblastoma [320-321]. MFH was well-tolarated by all patients in both studies with promising results.

Magnetic Resonance Imaging

MRI is a noninvasive imaging modality capable of providing high-resolution anatomical images which allows the differentiation between malignant and healthy tissues. SPIONs are excellent contrast MRI agents because of their T2* property with excellent sensitivity in T2* and T2 weighted images, as compared to other MRI agents [322, 323]. After iv administration, SPIONs larger than 50nm in diameter are rapidly sequested by hepatic and splenic macrophages, resulting in hypointense T2 weighted images of the normal tissue. In the liver, the lack of Kupffer cells in the tumour aids the differentiation between healthy and malignant regions [324-326] thus proving clinically useful in the diagnosis of liver tumours and metastases [328-329]. On the contrary, SPIONs of small sizes (diameter lower than 50nm) avoid massive uptake by macrophages of the liver and spleen, resulting in longer circulation. In fact, these SPIONs exhibit the ability to escape systemic circulation and gain access into deeper pathological tissues before uptake by local inflammatory macrophages [330-332]. Moreover, SPIONs have been successfully used for the detection of lymph node metastases [333-340], imaging of atherosclerotic plaques on the arterial wall [341-345], imaging of the inflammatory response in CNS disorders (ischaemic stroke lesions, cerebral inflammation, multiple sclerosis) [346-351], imaging of macrophage infiltration in transplanted organs [352, 353] and imaging of macrophage infiltration in knee joints [354-359].

Tissue Enginnering

Tissue engineering deals with the construction of biocompatible microstructured two or three dimensional scaffolds on which the cells can undergo attachment, growth, differentiation and proliferation. Cell cononisation can take place either *ex vivo* or *in vivo* [360].

MCLs employed for tissue engineering have been used to promote the adhesion of human aortic endothelial cells (HAECs) onto a rat hepatocyte layer [361]. Scaffolds for tissue engineering should be biocompatible and non-toxic. A crucial point is to reach a high cell number with sufficient packaging of the cells at the interior of the scaffold and this has been adressed by loading the cells with MCLs [362] or chitosan loaded MNPs [363], hydrating the scaffold with the suspension of the cells and applying a magnetic field. The magnetic field intensity has been found to have a positive influence on the depth of the cell seeding into the scaffold. Furhter, MCLs surface-functionalised with RGD sequence have been used as a cell-adhesion promoter for facilitating efficient cell patterning under the infuelnce of a magnetic field in order for the manufactured tissue to resemble normal tissue physiology [364]. Magnetic force-based tissue engineering also represents a promising approach for vascular tissue construction [365].

Encouraging results have been reported concerning the vascular grafting of human tissues such as human smooth muscle cells and dermal fibroblasts. The deposition of MCL-labelled cells onto a tubular vascular scaffold made of porcine decellularized common carotid artery, has been successfully achieved using an external magnetic field [366]. Also, MCLs have been employed to build three-dimensional tissues without scaffolds for bone-tissue reconstruction [367-368]. In another study, Femuroxide-loaded rabbit bone marrow derived mesenchymal cells were used to fill the bone defect, using interconnected porous calcium hydroxyapatite ceramic as substrate [369]. This technique could potentially treat bone defects and fractures. Another report revealed successful magnetic guidance of the intra-articularly injected IONP-labelled bone marrow-derived mesenchymal stem cells to osteochondral defects in a rabbit model [370]. Scaffold-free multilayered three-dimensional functional cardiomyocyte sheets have also been constructed using MCLs and magnetic field for heart-tissue engineering [371].

Conclusion

Magnetic nanoparticles represent a promising tool in personalized medicine due to their intrinsic characteristics and engineering susceptibility. Their utilization has allowed the advancement of medical imaging, drug delivery, cancer therapy and magnetic hyperthermia and has also broadened the frontiers of emerging fields such as gene delivery, tissue engineering, cell tracking and bioseparation. However, there are certain properties of MNPs that amplify their toxicity and these should be taken into careful consideration and investigated further in order to balance the benefit to risk ratio in biomedical applications. Moreover, the use of MNPs for drug-delivery applications is somewhat limited by the complexity involved in the setup of external magnetic fields and the distance between the target site and the magnetic field.

Various pre-clinical and clinical trials are currently in progress aiming to investigate the potential of different magnetic nanosystems for pharmaceutical and biomedical applications.

References

[1] King, J. G.; Williams, W.; Wilkinson, C. D. W.; McVitie, S.; Chapman, J. N. *Geophys. Res. Lett.* 1996, 23, 2847.

[2] Rishton, A.; Lu, Y.; Altman, R. A.; Marley, A. C.; Bian Hahnes, C.; Viswanathan, R.; Xiao, G.; Gallagher, W. J.; Parkin, S. S. P. *Microelectron. Eng.* 1997, 35, 249.

[3] Lee, C. S.; Lee, H.; Westervelt, R. M. *Appl. Phys. Lett.* 2001, 79, 3308.

[4] Mathur, S.; Barth, S.; Werner, U.; Hernandez-Ramirez, F.; Romano-Rodriguez, A. *Adv. Mater.* 2008, 20, 1550.

[5] Narayanan, K. B.; Sakthivel, N. Adv. *Colloid Interface Sci.* 2010, 156, 1.

[6] Moon, J. W.; Roh, Y.; Lauf, R. J.; Vali, H.; Yeary, L. W.; Phelps, T. J. *J. Microbiol. Methods* 2007, 70, 150.

[7] Moon, J. W.; Rawn, C. J.; Rondinone, A. J.; Love, L. J.; Roh, Y.; Everett, S. M.; Lauf, R. J.; Phelps, T. J. *J. Ind. Microbiol. Biotechnol.* 2010, 37, 1023.

[8] da Costa, G. M.; de Grave, E.; de Bakker, P. M. A.; Vandenberghe, R. E. J. *Solid State Chem.* 1994, 113, 405.

[9] Itoh, H.; Sugimoto, T. J. *Colloid Interface Sci.* 2003, 265, 283.

[10] Amemiya, Y.; Arakaki, A.; Staniland, S. S.; Tanaka, T.; Matsunaga, T. *Biomaterials* 2007, 28, 5381.

[11] Vereda, F.; Rodríguez-Gonzalez, B.; de Vicente, J.; Hidalgo- Álvarez, R. J. *Colloid Interface Sci.* 2008, 318, 520.

[12] Massart, R. *IEEE Trans. Magn.* 1981, 17, 1247.

[13] Wu, J. H.; Ko, S. P.; Liu, H. L.; Kim, S.; Ju, J. S.; Kim, Y. K. *Mater. Lett.* 2007, 61, 3124.

[14] Khollam, Y. B.; Dhage, S. R.; Potdar, H. S.; Deshpande, S. B.; Bakare, P. P.; Kulkarni, S. D.; Date, S. K. *Mater. Lett.* 2002, 56, 571.

[15] Chen, F.; Gao, Q.; Hong, G.; Ni, J. J. *Magn. Magn. Mater.* 2008, 320, 1775.

[16] Salazar-Alvarez, G.; Muhammed, M.; Zagorodni, A. A. *Chem. Eng. Sci.* 2006, 61, 4625.

[17] Cabrera, L.; Gutierrez, S.; Menendes, N.; Morales, M. P.; Herrasti, P. *Electrochem. Acta* 2008, 53, 3436.

[18] Marques, R. F. C.; Garcia, C.; Lecante, P.; Ribeiro, J. L.; Noé, L.; Silva, N. J. O.; Amaral, V. S.; Millan, A.; Verelst, M. J. *Magn. Magn. Mater.* 2008, 320, 2311.

[19] Gonzalez-Carreño, T.; Morales, M. P.; Gracia, M.; Serna, C. *J. Mater. Lett.* 1993, 18, 151.

[20] Strobel, R.; Pratsinis, S. E. *Adv. Powder Technol.* 2009, 20, 190.

[21] Enomoto, N.; Akagi, J.; Nakagawa, Z. *Ultrason. Sonochem.* 1996, 3, S97.

[22] Dang, F.; Enomoto, N.; Hojo, J.; Enpuku, K. *Ultrason. Sonochem.* 2009, 16, 649.

[23] Eckert, C. A.; Knutson, B. L.; Debenedetti, P. G. *Nature* 1996, 383, 313.

[24] Teng Lam, U.; Mammucari, R.; Suzuki, K.; Foster, N. R. *Ind. Eng. Chem. Res.* 2008, 47, 599.

[25] Breulmann, M.; Colfen, H.; Hentze, H. P.; Antonietti, M.; Walsh, D.; Mann, S. *Adv. Mater.* 1998, 10, 237.

[26] Bakar, M. A.; Tan, W. L.; Bakar, N. H. H. A. J. *Magn. Magn. Mater.* 2007, 314, 1.

[27] Liu, X. M.; Yang, G.; Fu, S. Y. *Mater. Sci. Eng.*, C 2007, 27, 750.

[28] Gunjakar, J. L.; More, A. M.; Shinde, V. R.; Lokhande, C. D. J. *Alloys Compd.* 2008, 465, 468.

[29] Naidek, K. P.; Bianconi, F.; da Rocha, T. C. R.; Zanchet, D.; Bonacin, J. A.; Novak, M. A.; Vaz, M. G. F.; Winnischofer, H. J. *Colloid Interface Sci.* 2011, 358, 39.

[30] Kim, S.; Shibata, E.; Sergiienko, R.; Nakamura, T. *Carbon* 2008, 46, 1523.

[31] Cao, H.; Huang, G.; Xuan, S.; Wu, Q.; Gu, F.; Li, C. *J. Alloys Compd.* 2008, 448, 272.

[32] Gupta, A. K.; Curtis, A. S. G. J. *Mater. Sci. Mater. Med.* 2004, 15, 493.
[33] Ma, D. L.; Guan, J. W.; Normandin, F.; Denommee, S.; Enright, G.; Veres, T.; Simard, B. *Chem. Mater.* 2006, 18, 1920.
[34] Chen, S.; Li, Y.; Guo, C.; Wang, J.; Ma, J.; Liang, X.; Yang, L. R.; Liu, H. Z. *Langmuir* 2007, 23, 12669.
[35] de Cuyper, M.; Soenen, S. J. H.; Coenegrachts, K.; Beek, L. T. *Anal. Biochem.* 2007, 367, 266.
[36] Liu, H.; Guo, J.; Jin, L.; Yang, W.; Wang, C. J. *Phys. Chem.* B 2008, 112, 3315.
[37] Sahoo, Y.; Pizem, H.; Fried, T.; Golodnitsky, D.; Burstein, L.; Sukenik, C. N.; Markovich, G. *Langmuir* 2001, 17, 7907.
[38] Kim, E. H.; Lee, H. S.; Kwak, B. K.; Kim, B. K. J. *Magn. Magn. Mater.* 2005, 289, 328.
[39] Woo, K.; Hong, J.; Ahn, J. P. J. *Magn. Magn. Mater.* 2005, 293, 177.
[40] Selim, K. M. K.; Ha, Y. S.; Kim, S. J.; Chang, Y.; Kim, T. J.; Lee, G. H.; Kang, I. K. *Biomaterials* 2007, 28, 710.
[41] Hodenius, M.; De Cuyper, M.; Desender, L.; Muller-Schulte, D.; Steigel, A.; Lueken, H. *Chem. Phys. Lipids* 2002, 120, 75.
[42] Roberts, D.; Zhu, W. L.; Fromenn, C. M.; Rosenzweig, Z. *J. Appl. Phys.* 2000, 87, 6208.
[43] Bautista, M. C.; Bomati-Miguel, O.; Morales, M. D.; Serna, C. J.; Veintemillas-Verdaguer, S. J. *Magn. Magn. Mater.* 2005, 293, 20.
[44] Morales, M. A.; Fitonelli, P. V.; Coaquira, J. A. H.; Rocha-Leao, M. H. M.; Diaz-Aguila, C.; Baggio-Saitovitch, E. M.; Rossi, A. M. *Mater. Sci. Eng.,* C 2008, 28, 253.
[45] Jia, Z.; Yujun, W.; Yangcheng, L.; Jingyu, M.; Guangsheng, L. *React. Funct. Polym.* 2006, 66, 1552.
[46] Shinkai, M. S.; Suzuki, M.; Iijima, S.; Kobayashi, T. *Biotechnol. Appl. Biochem.* 1994, 21, 125.
[47] Huth, S.; Lausier, J.; Gersting, S. W.; Rudolph, C.; Plank, C.; Welsch, U.; Rosenecker, J. J. *Gene Med.* 2004, 6, 923.
[48] Duran, J. D. G.; Arias, J. L.; Gallardo, V.; Delgado, A. V. J. *Pharm. Sci.* 2008, 97, 2948.
[49] Zhang, M.; Ferrari, M. J. *Biomed. Microdev.* 1998, 1, 81.
[50] Gref, R.; Luck, M.; Quellec, P.; Marchand, M.; Dellacherie, E.; Harnisch, S.; Blunk, T.; Müller, R. H. *Colloids Surf.*, B 2000, 18, 301.
[51] Shang, H.; Chang, W. S.; Kan, S.; Majetich, S. A.; Lee, G. U. *Langmuir* 2006, 22, 2516.

[52] Shen, T.; Weissleder, R.; Papisov, M.; Bogdanov, A., Jr.; Brady, T. J. *Magn. Reson. Med.* 1993, 29, 599.

[53] Josephson, L.; Tung, C. H.; Moore, A.; Weissleder, R. *Bioconjugate Chem.* 1999, 10, 186.

[54] Corot, C.; Robert, P.; Idee, J. M.; Port, M. *Adv. Drug Delivery Rev.* 2006, 58, 1471.

[55] Lu, A. H.; Salabas, E. L.; Schuth, F. *Angew. Chem., Int. Ed.* 2007, 46, 1222.

[56] Seo, W. S.; Lee, J. H.; Sun, X.; Suzuki, Y.; Mann, D.; Liu, Z.; Terashima, M.; Yang, P. C.; McConnell, M. V.; Nishimura, D. G.; Dai, H. *Nat. Mater.* 2006, 5, 971.

[57] Lu, Y.; Yin, Y. D.; Mayers, B. T.; Xia, Y. N. *Nano Lett.* 2002, 2, 183.

[58] Tan, W. H.; Wang, K. M.; He, X. X.; Zhao, X. J.; Drake, T.; Wang, L.; Bagwe, R. P. *Med. Res. Rev.* 2004, 24, 621.

[59] Tada, D. B.; Vono, L. L. R.; Duarte, D. L.; Itri, R.; Kiyohara, P. .; Baptista, M. S.; Rossi, L. M. *Langmuir* 2007, 23, 8194.

[60] Bi, S.; Wei, X.; Li, N.; Lei, Z. *Mater. Lett.* 2008, 62, 2963. Peng, S.; Wang, C.; Xie, J.; Sun, S. J. *Am. Chem. Soc.* 2006, 128, 10676.

[61] Qiang, Y.; Antony, J.; Sharma, A.; Nutting, J.; Sikes, D.; Meyer, D. J. *Nanoparticle Res.* 2006, 8, 489.

[62] Tartaj, P.; Gonzalez-Carreño, T.; Serna, C. J. *Langmuir* 2002, 18, 4556.

[63] Arruebo, M.; Galan, M.; Navascues, N.; Tellez, C.; Marquina, C.; Ibarra, M. R.; Santamaría, *J. Chem. Mater.* 2006, 18, 1911.

[64] Arruebo, M.; Fernandez-Pacheco, R.; Hirsuta, S.; Arbiol, J.; Ibarra, M. R.; Santamaría, *J. Nanotechnology* 2006, 17, 4057.

[65] Carja, G.; Chiriac, H.; Lupu, N. J. *Magn. Magn. Mater.* 2007, 311, 26.

[66] Fernandez-Pacheco, R.; Arruebo, M.; Marquina, C.; Ibarra, R.; Arbiol, J.; Santamaría, *J. Nanotechnology* 2006, 17, 1188.

[67] Liang, Y. Y.; Zhang, L. M.; Jiang, W.; Li, W. *ChemPhysChem* 2007, 8, 2367.

[68] Saravanan, M.; Bhaskar, K.; Mahajaran, G.; Pillai, K. S. *Int. J. Pharm.* 2004, 283, 71.

[69] Alexiou, C.; Schmid, R. J.; Jurgons, R.; Kremer, M.; Wanner, G.; Bergemann, C.; Huenges, E.; Nawroth, T.; Arnold, W.; Parak, F. G. *Eur. Biophys. J.* 2006, 35, 446.

[70] Kim, D. H.; Lee, S. H.; Im, K. H.; Kim, K. N.; Kim, K. M.; Shim, I. B.; Lee, M. H.; Lee, Y. K. *Curr. Appl. Phys.* 2006, 6, e242.

[71] Ma, H. L.; Xu, Y. F.; Qi, X. R.; Maitani, Y.; Nagai, T. *Int. J. Pharm.* 2008, 354, 217.

[72] Viota, J. L.; Delgado, A. V.; Arias, J. L.; Duran, J. D. G. J. *Colloid Interface Sci.* 2008, 324, 199.

[73] Lin, P. C.; Chou, P. H.; Chen, S. H.; Liao, H. K.; Wang, K. Y.; Chen, Y. J.; Lin, C. C. *Small* 2006, 2, 485.

[74] Balakrishnan, S.; Bonder, M. J.; Hadjipanayis, G. C. J. *Magn. Magn. Mater.* 2009, 321, 117.

[75] Gomez-Lopera, S. A.; Plaza, R. C.; Delgado, A. V. *J. Colloid Interface* Sci. 2001, 240, 40.

[76] Gomez-Lopera, S. A.; Arias, J. L.; Gallardo, V.; Delgado, A. V. *Langmuir* 2006, 22, 2816.

[77] Hamoudeh, M.; Faraj, A. A.; Canet-Soulas, E.; Bessueille, F.; Leonard, D.; Fessi, H. *Int. J. Pharm.* 2007, 338, 248.

[78] Kumagai, M.; Imai, Y.; Nakamura, T.; Yamasaki, Y.; Sekino, M.; Ueno, S.; Hanaoka, K.; Kikuchi, K.; Nagano, T.; Kaneko, E.; Shimokado, K.; Kataoka, K. *Colloids Surf.,* B 2007, 56, 174.

[79] Fan, Q. L.; Neoh, K. G.; Kang, E. T.; Shuter, B.; Wang, S. C. *Biomaterials* 2007, 28, 5426.

[80] Ren, J.; Hong, H. Y.; Ren, T. B.; Teng, X. R. *Mater. Lett.* 2005, 59, 2655.

[81] Nasongkla, N.; Bey, E.; Ren, J. M.; Ai, H.; Khemtong, C.; Guthi, J. S.; Chin, S. F.; Sherry, A. D.; Boothman, D. A.; Gao, J. M. *Nano Lett.* 2006, 6, 2427.

[82] Okassa, L. N.; Marchais, H.; Douziech-Eyrolles, L.; Cohen-Jonathan, S.; Soucé, M.; Dubois, P.; Chourpa, I. *Int. J. Pharm.* 2005, 302, 187.

[83] Okassa, L. N.; Marchais, H.; Douziech-Eyrolles, L.; Hervé, K.; Cohen-Jonathan, S.; Munnier, E.; Soucé, M.; Linassier, C.; Dubois, P.; Chourpa, I. *Eur. J. Pharm. Biopharm.* 2007, 67, 31.

[84] Liu, X.; Kaminski, M. D.; Chen, H.; Torno, M.; Taylor, L.; Rosengart, A. J. *J. Controlled Release* 2007, 119, 52.

[85] Holgado, M. A.; Álvarez-Fuentes, J.; Fernandez-Arevalo, M.; Arias, J. L. *Curr. Drug Targets* 2011, 12, 1096.

[86] Perez-Artacho, B.; Gallardo, V.; Ruiz, M. A.; Arias, J. L. *J. Nanopart. Res.* 2012, 14, 768.

[87] Arias, J. L.; Gallardo, V.; Gomez-Lopera, S. A.; Delgado, A. V. *J. Biomed. Nanotechol.* 2005, 1, 214.

[88] Arias, J. L.; Gallardo, V.; Ruiz, M. A.; Delgado, A. V. *Eur. J. Pharm. Biopharm.* 2008, 69, 54.

[89] Arias, J. L.; Ruiz, M. A.; Gallardo, V.; Delgado, A. V. *J. Controlled Release* 2008, 125, 50.
[90] Arias, J. L.; Linares-Molinero, F.; Gallardo, V.; Delgado, A. V. Eur. *J. Pharm. Sci.* 2008, 33, 252.
[91] Yang, J.; Lee, H.; Hyung, W.; Park, S. B.; Haam, S. *J. Microencapsulation* 2006, 23, 203.
[92] Arias, J. L.; Saez-Fernandez, E.; Lopez-Viota, M.; Biedma-Ortiz, R. A.; Ruiz, M. A. *Med. Chem.* 2012, 8, 516.
[93] Wang, S. F.; Tan, Y. M. Anal. Bioanal. Chem. 2007, 387, 703. Arias, J. L.; Reddy, L. H.; Couvreur, P. J. *Mater. Chem*. 2012, 22, 7622.
[94] Santos, D. P.; Ruiz, M. A.; Gallardo, V.; Zanoni, M. V. B.; Arias, J. L. *J. Nanoparticle Res*. 2011, 13, 4311.
[95] Flesch, C.; Bourgeat-Lami, E.; Mornet, S.; Duguet, E.; Delaite, C.; Dumas, P. *J. Polym. Sci., Part A: Polym. Chem*. 2005, 43, 3221.
[96] Yang, J.; Park, S. B.; Yoon, H. G.; Huh, Y. M.; Haam, S. *Int. J. Pharm*. 2006, 324, 185.
[97] Arias, J. L.; Lopez-Viota, M.; Ruiz, M. A.; Lopez-Viota, J.; Delgado, A. V. *Int. J. Pharm*. 2007, 339, 237.
[98] Arias, J. L.; Lopez-Viota, M.; Delgado, A. V.; Ruiz, M. A. *Colloids Surf.,* B 2010, 77, 111.
[99] Yang, C.; Guan, Y.; Xing, J.; Liu, H. *Langmuir* 2008, 24, 9006.
[100] Gass, J.; Poddar, P.; Almand, J.; Srinath, S.; Srikanth, H. *Adv. Funct. Mater.* 2006, 16, 71.
[101] Yuan, J. J.; Armes, S. P.; Takabayashi, Y.; Prassides, K.; Leite, C. A. P.; Galembeck, F.; Lewis, A. L. *Langmuir* 2006, 22, 10989.
[102] Dey, T. J. *Nanosci. Nanotechnol*. 2006, 6, 2479.
[103] Hu, S. H.; Liu, T. Y.; Liu, D. M.; Chen, S. Y. J. *Controlled Release* 2007, 121, 181.
[104] Boissiere, M.; Allouche, J.; Brayner, R.; Chaneac, C.; Livage, J.;Coradin, T. J. *Nanosci. Nanotechnol.* 2007, 7, 4649.
[105] Phanapavudhikul, P.; Shen, S.; Ng, W. K.; Tan, R. B. H. *Drug Delivery* 2008, 15, 177.
[106] Lee, J.; Isobe, T.; Senna, M. *J. Colloid Interface Sci.* 1996, 177,490.
[107] Mikhaylova, M.; Jo, Y. S.; Kim, D. K.; Bobrysheva, N.; Anderson, Y.; Eriksson, T.; Osmolowsky, M.; Semenov, V.; Muhammed, M. *Hyperfine Interact.* 2004, 156, 257.
[108] Mikhaylova, M.; Kim, D. K.; Bobrysheva, N.; Osmolowsky, M.; Semenov, V.; Tsakalakos, T.; Muhammed, M. *Langmuir* 2004, 20, 2472.

[109] Arias, J. L.; Clares, B.; Morales, M. E.; Gallardo, V.; Ruiz, M. A. Curr. *Drug Targets* 2011, 12, 1151.
[110] Martina, M. S.; Fortin, J. P.; Menager, C.; Clement, O.; Barratt,G.; Gabrielle-Madelmont, C.; Gazeau, F.; Cabuil, V.; Lesieur, S. J. *Am. Chem. Soc.* 2005, 127, 10676.
[111] Hergt, R.; Dutz, S.; Müller, R.; Zeisberger, M. *J. Phys. Cond. Mater.* 2006, 18, S2919.
[112] Lang, C.; Schüler, D.; Faivre, D. *Macromol. Biosci.* 2007, 7, 144.
[113] Xiang, L.; Wei, J.; Jianbo, S.; Guili, W.; Feng, G.; Ying, L. *Lett. Appl. Microbiol.* 2007, 45, 75.
[114] Bulte, J. W. M.; de Cuyper, M.; Despres, D.; Frank, J. A. *J. Magn. Magn. Mater.* 1999, 194, 204.
[115] Yoshino, T.; Hirabe, H.; Takahashi, M.; Kuhara, M.; Takeyama, H.; Matsunaga, T. *Biotechnol. Bioeng.* 2008, 101, 470.
[116] Huang, X.; Bronstein, L. M.; Retrum, J.; Dufort, C.; Tsvetkova, I.; Aniagyei, S.; Stein, B.; Stucky, G.; McKenna, B.; Remmes, N.; Baxter, D.; Kao, C. C.; Dragnea, B. *Nano Lett.* 2007, 7, 2407.
[117] Di Marco, M.; Port, M.; Couvreur, P.; Dubernet, C.; Ballirano, P.; Sadun, C. J. *Am. Chem. Soc.* 2006, 128, 10054.
[118] Weissleder, R.; Reimer, P.; Lee, A. S.; Wittenberg, J.; Brady, T. *Am. J. Roentgenol.* 1990, 155, 1161.
[119] Weissleder, R.; Elizondo, G.; Wittenberg, J.; Rabito, C. A.; Bengele, H. H.; Josephson, L. *Radiology* 1990, 175, 489.
[120] Moeser, G. D.; Green, W. H.; Laibinis, P. E.; Linse, P.; Hatton, T. A. *Langmuir* 2004, 20, 5223.
[121] Sadun, C.; Bucci, R.; Magri, A. L. J. *Am. Chem. Soc.* 2002, 124, 3036.
[122] Miser, D. E.; Shin, E. J.; Hajaligol, M. R.; Rasouli, F. *Appl. Catal.*, A 2004, 258, 7.
[123] Brice-Profeta, S.; Arrio, M. A.; Tronc, E.; Menguy, N.; Letard, I.; Cartier dit Moulin, C.; Nogues, M.; Chaneac, C.; Jolivet, J. P.; Sainctavit, *Ph. J. Magn. Magn. Mater.* 2005, 288, 354.
[124] Yee, C.; Kataby, G.; Ulman, A.; Prozorov, T.; White, H.; King, A.; Rafailovich, M.; Sokolov, J.; Gedanken, A. *Langmuir* 1999, 15, 7111.
[125] Roger, J.; Pons, J. N.; Massart, R.; Halbreich, A.; Bacri, J. C. *Eur. Phys. J.: Appl. Phys.* 1999, 5, 321.
[126] Nooney, M. G.; Corneille, J. S.; Murrell, T. S.; Lin, X. F.; Hossner, L. R.; Chusuei, C. C.; Goodman, D. W. *Langmuir* 1998, 14, 2750.
[127] Neuberger, T.; Schöpf, B.; Hotmann, H.; Hofmann, M.; von Rechenberg, B. J. *Magn. Magn. Mater.* 2005, 293, 483.

[128] Weissleder, R.; Bogdanov, A.; Neuwelt, E. A.; Papisov, M. *Adv.Drug Delivery Rev.* 1995, 16, 321.
[129] Schütt, W.; Grüttner, C.; Hafeli, U.; Zborowski, M.; Teller, J.;Putzar, H.; Schümichen, C. *Hybridoma* 1997, 16, 109.
[130] Lin, X. M.; Samia, A. C. S. J. *Magn. Magn. Mater.* 2006, 305,100.
[131] Janssen, J. J. M.; Baltussen, J. J. M.; van Gelder, A. P.;Perenboom, J. A. A. J. J. Phys. D, *Appl. Phys.* 1990, 23, 1455.
[132] Ortega-Vinuesa, J. L.; Martin-Rodriguez, A.; Hidalgo-Alvarez, R. *J. Colloid Interface Sci.* 1996, 184, 259.
[133] Romero-Cano, M. S.; Martín-Rodríguez, A.; de las Nieves, F. *J. Langmuir* 2001, 17, 3505.
[134] Valle-Delgado, J. J.; Molina-Bolıvar, J. A.; Galisteo-Gonzalez,F.; Galvez-Ruiz, M. *J. Colloid Polym. Sci.* 2003, 81, 708.
[135] Hunter, R. J. *Foundations of Colloid Science*, 2nd ed.; Clarendon Press: Oxford, U.K., 2001.
[136] Thode, K.; Muller, R. H.; Kresse, M. *J. Pharm. Sci.* 2000, 89,1317.
[137] Blunk, T.; Hochstrasser, D. F.; Sanchez, J.; Müller, B. W.; Müller, R. H. *Electrophoresis* 1993, 14, 1382.
[138] Borchard, G.; Kreuter, J. J. *Drug Targeting* 1993, 1, 15.
[139] Borchard, G.; Kreuter, J. *Pharm. Res.* 1996, 13, 1055.
[140] Armstrong, T. I.; Davies, M. C.; Illum, L. J. *Drug Targeting1997*, 4, 389.
[141] Arruebo, M.; Fernandez-Pacheco, R.; Ibarra, M. R.; Santamaría, J. *Nano Today* 2007, 2, 22.
[142] Decuzzi, P.; Ferrari, M. *Biomaterials* 2006, 27, 5307.
[143] Gref, R.; Minamitake, Y.; Peracchia, M. T.; Trubetskoy, V.;Torchilin, V.; Langer, R. *Science* 1994, 263, 1600.
[144] Farokhzad, O. C.; Cheng, J.; Teply, B. A.; Sherifi, I.; Jon, S.;Kantoff, P. W.; Richie, J. P.; Langer, R. *Proc. Natl. Acad. Sci. USA.*2006, 103, 6315.
[145] Matsumura, Y. Adv. *Drug Delivery Rev.* 2008, 60, 899.
[146] Oussoren, C.; Storm, G. J. *Liposome Res.* 1999, 9, 349.
[147] Coins, B.; Phillips, W. T.; Klipper, R. J. *Liposome Res.* 1998, 8,265.
[148] Laverman, P.; Carstens, M. G.; Boerman, O. C.; Dams, E. M.;Oyen, W. J. G.; van Rooijen, N.; Corstens, F. M.; Storm, G. J. *Pharmacol. Exp. Ther.* 2001, 298, 607.
[149] Ishida, T.; Kiwada, H. *Int. J. Pharm.* 2008, 354, 56.
[150] Ishida, T.; Harada, M.; Wang, X. Y.; Ichihara, M.; Irimura, K.; Kiwada, H. J. *Controlled Release* 2005, 105, 305.

[151] Ishida, T.; Atobe, K.; Wang, X.; Kiwada, H. J. *Controlled Release* 2006, 115, 251.

[152] Ishihara, T.; Takeda, M.; Sakamoto, H.; Kimoto, A.; Kobayashi,C.; Takasaki, N.; Yuki, K.; Tanaka, K.; Takenaga, M.; Igarashi, R.; Maeda, T.; Yamakawa, N.; Okamoto, Y.; Otsuka, M.; Ishida, T.; Kiwada, H.; Mizushima, Y.; Mizushima, T. *Pharm. Res*. 2009, 26, 2270.

[153] Ishihara, T.; Maeda, T.; Sakamoto, H.; Takasaki, N.; Shigyo, M.; Ishida, T.; Kiwada, H.; Mizushima, Y.; Mizushima, T. *Biomacromolecules* 2010, 11, 2700.

[154] Maeda, H. Adv. *Enzyme Reg*. 2001, 41, 189.

[155] Maeda, H. *Bioconjugate Chem*. 2010, 21, 797.

[156] Senyei, A.; Widder, K.; Czerlinski, G. J. *Appl. Phys*. 1978, 49,3578.

[157] Dobson, J. *Drug Dev. Res*. 2006, 67, 55.

[158] Fang, C.; Shi, B.; Pei, Y. Y.; Hong, M. H.; Wu, J.; Chen, H. Z. *Eur. J. Pharm. Sci*. 2006, 27, 27.

[159] Majumdar, S.; Zoghbi, S. S.; Gore, J. C. *Invest. Radiol*. 1990, 25,771.

[160] Varallyay, P.; Nesbit, G.; Muldoon, L. L.; Nixon, R. R.; Delashaw, J.; Cohen, J. I.; Petrillo, A.; Rink, D.; Neuwelt, E. A. *Am. J. Neuroradiol*. 2002, 23, 510.

[161] Bourrinet, P.; Bengele, H. H.; Bonnemain, B.; Dencausse, A.; Idee, J. M.; Jacobs, P. M.; Lewis, J. M. *Invest. Radiol*. 2006, 41, 313.

[162] Chouly, C.; Pouliquen, D.; Lucet, I.; Jeune, J. J.; Jallet, P. *J. Microencapsulation* 1996, 13, 245.

[163] Maaßen, S.; Fattal, E.; Müller, R. H.; Couvreur, P. *STP Pharma Sci*. 1993, 3, 11.

[164] Iannone, A.; Magin, R. L.; Walczack, T.; Federico, M.; Swartz,H. M.; Tomasi, A.; Vannini, V. *Magn. Reson. Med*. 1991, 22, 435.

[165] Moghimi, M. M.; Hunter, A. C.; Murray, J. C. *Pharmacol. Rev*. 2001, 53, 283.

[166] Weissleder, R.; Bogdanov, A.; Neuwelt, E. A.; Papisov, M. *Adv. Drug Delivery Rev*. 1995, 16, 321.

[167] Fujita, T.; Nishikawa, M.; Ohtsubo, Y.; Ohno, J.; Takakura, Y.;Sezaki, H.; Hashida, M. J. *Drug Targeting* 1994, 2, 157.

[168] Papisov, M. I.; Bogdanov, A.; Schaffer, B.; Nossiff, N.; Shen, T.;Weissleder, R.; Brady, T. J. J. *Magn. Magn. Mater*. 1993, 122, 383.

[169] Kwon, J. T.; Hwang, S. K.; Jin, H.; Kim, D. S.; Minai-Tehrani,A.; Yoon, H. J.; Choi, M.; Yoon, T. J.; Han, D. Y.; Kang, Y. W.; Yoon,B. I.; Lee, J. K.; Cho, M. H. J. *Occup. Health* 2008, 50, 1.

[170] Kim, J. S.; Yoon, T. J.; Yu, K. N.; Kim, B. G.; Park, S. J.; Kim,H. W.; Lee, K. H.; Park, S. B.; Lee, J. K.; Cho, M. H. *Toxicol. Sci.* 2006,89, 338.

[171] Choi, H. S.; Liu, W.; Misra, P.; Tanaka, E.; Zimmer, J. P.; Ipe,B. I.; Bawendi, M. G.; Frangioni, J. V. *Nat. Biotechnol.* 2007, 25, 1165.

[172] Briley-Saebo, K.; Bjørnerud, A.; Grant, D.; Ahlstrom, H.; Berg,T.; Kindberg, G. M. *Cell Tissue Res.* 2004, 316, 315.

[173] Briley-Saebø, K.; Hustvedt, S. O.; Haldorsen, A.; Bjørnerud, A.J. *Magn. Reson. Imaging* 2004, 20, 622.

[174] Dupas, B.; Berreur, M.; Rohanizadeh, R.; Bonnemain, B.;Meflah, K.; Pradal, G. *Biol Cell.* 1999, 91, 195.

[175] Raynal, I.; Prigent, P.; Peyramaure, S.; Najid, A.; Rebuzzi, C.; Corot, C. *Invest. Radiol.* 2004, 39, 56.

[176] Schulze, E.; Ferrucci, J. T., Jr.; Poss, K.; Lapointe, L.;Bogdanova, A.; Weissleder, R. *Invest Radiol.* 1995, 30, 604.

[177] Simioni, A. R.; Martins, O. P.; Lacava, Z. G.; Azevedo, R. B.;Lima, E. C.; Lacava, B. M.; Morais, P. C.; Tedesco, A. C. *J. Nanosci. Nanotechnol.* 2006, 6, 2413.

[178] Müller, K.; Skepper, J. N.; Posfai, M.; Trivedi, R.; Howarth, S.; Corot, C.; Lancelot, E.; Thompson, P. W.; Brown, A. P.; Gillard, J. H. *Biomaterials* 2007, 28, 1629.

[179] Karlsson, H. L.; Gustafsson, J.; Cronholm, P.; Möller, L. *Toxicol. Lett.* 2009, 188, 112.

[180] Mahmoudi, M.; Simchi, A.; Imani, M.; Shokrgozar, M. A.;Milani, A. S.; Hafeli, U. O.; Stroeve, P. *Colloids Surf B Biointerfaces* 2010, 75, 300.

[181] Pisanic, T. R., II; Blackwell, J. D.; Shubayev, V. I.; Fiñones, R. R.; Jin, S. *Biomaterials* 2007, 28, 2572.

[182] de Freitas, E. R.; Soares, P. R.; Santos, R. P.; dos Santos, R. L.;da Silva, J. R.; Porfirio, E. P.; Bao, S. N.; Lima, E. C.; Morais, P. C.; Guillo, L. A. *J. Nanosci. Nanotechnol.* 2008, 8, 2385.

[183] Weissleder, R.; Stark, D. D.; Engelstad, B. L.; Bacon, B. R.;Compton, C. C.; White, D. L.; Jacobs, P.; Lewis, J. *Am. J. Roentgenol.*1989, 152, 167.

[184] Klausner, R. D.; Ronault, T. A.; Harford, J. B. *Cell* 1993, 72, 19.

[185] Elias, A.; Tsourkas, A. *Hematology Am. Soc. Hematol. Educ.Program* 2009, 2009, 720.

[186] Glickstein, H.; El, R. B.; Link, G.; Breuer, W.; Konijn, A. M.; Hershko, C.; Nick, H.; Cabantchik, Z. I. *Blood* 2006, 108, 3195.

[187] Jain, T. K.; Reddy, M. K.; Morales, M. A.; Leslie-Pelecky, D. L.;Labhasetwar, V. *Mol. Pharmaceutics* 2008, 5, 316.

[188] Lübbe, A. S.; Bergemann, C.; Riess, H.; Schriever, F.; Reichardt, P.; Possinger, K.; Matthias, M.; Dörken, B.; Herrmann,F.; Gürtler, R.; Hohenberger, P.; Haas, N.; Sohr, R.; Sander, B.; Lemke, A. J.; Ohlendorf, D.; Huhnt, W.; Huhn, D. *Cancer Res.* 1996,56, 4686.

[189] Lemke, A. J.; Senfft von Pilsach, M. I.; Lübbe, A.; Bergemann, C.; Riess, H.; Felix, R. *Eur. Radiol.* 2004, 14, 1949.

[190] Reimer, P.; Balzer, T. *Eur. Radiol.* 2003, 13, 1266.

[191] Reimer, P.; Marx, C.; Rummeny, E. J.; Müller, M.; Lentschig, M.; Balzer, T.; Dietl, K. H.; Sulkowski, U.; Berns, T.; Shamsi, K.;Peters, P. E. J. *Magn. Reson. Imaging* 1997, 7, 945.

[192] Kopp, A. F.; Laniado, M.; Dammann, F.; Stern, W.; Grönewaller, E.; Balzer, T.; Schimpfky, C.; Claussen, C. D. *Radiology* 1997, 204, 749.

[193] Kehagias, D. T.; Gouliamos, A. D.; Smyrniotis, V.; Vlahos, L. J.J. *Magn. Reson. Imaging* 2001, 14, 595.

[194] Muldoon, L. L.; Sandor, M.; Pinkston, K. E.; Neuwelt, E. A. *Neurosurgery* 2005, 57, 785.

[195] Aillon, K. L.; Xie, Y.; El-Gendy, N.; Berkland, C. J.; Forrest, M.L. Adv. *Drug Delivery Rev.* 2009, 61, 457.

[196] Alexis, F.; Pridgen, E.; Molnar, L. K.; Farokhzad, O. C. *Mol. Pharmaceutics* 2008, 5, 505.

[197] Lacava, Z. G. M.; Azevedo, R. B.; Martins, E. V.; Lacava, L. M.;Freitas, M. L. L.; Garcia, V. A. P.; Rehbula, C. A.; Lemos, A. P. C.;Sousa, M. H.; Tourinho, F. A.; Da Silva, M. F.; Morais, P. C. J. *Magn. Magn. Mater.* 1999, 201, 431.

[198] Yu, Z.; Xiaoliang, W.; Xuman, W.; Hong, X.; Hongchen, G. J. *Biomed. Mater. Res.* 2008, 85, 582.

[199] Kingsley, J. D.; Dou, H.; Morehead, J.; Rabinow, B.;Gendelman, H. E.; Destache, C. J. J. *Neuroimmune Pharmacol.* 2006,1, 340.

[200] Couvreur, P.; Vauthier, C. *Pharm. Res.* 2006, 23, 1417.

[201] Arias, J. L. *Mini-Rev. Med. Chem.* 2011, 11, 1.

[202] Ibrahim, A.; Couvreur, P.; Roland, M.; Speiser, P. J. *Pharm.Pharmacol.* 1983, 35, 59.

[203] Gallo, J. M.; Gupta, P. K.; Hung, C. T.; Perrier, D. G. J. *Pharm.Sci.* 1989, 78, 190.

[204] Gallo, J. M.; Hafeli, U. *Cancer Res.* 1997, 57, 3063.

[205] Alexiou, C.; Schmidt, A.; Klein, R.; Hulin, P.; Bergemann, C. J. *Magn. Magn. Mater.* 2002, 252, 363.

[206] Alexiou, C.; Jurgons, R.; Schmid, R. J.; Bergemann, C.; Henke,J.; Erhardt, W.; Huenges, E.; Parak, F. J. *Drug Targeting* 2003, 11, 139.

[207] Alexiou, C.; Jurgons, R.; Schmid, R.; Hilpert, A.; Bergemann,C.; Parak, F.; Iro, H. J. *Magn. Magn. Mater.* 2005, 293, 389.
[208] Kohler, N.; Sun, C.; Wang, J.; Zhang, M. Q. *Langmuir* 2005,21, 8858.
[209] Gupta, R.; Bajpai, A. K. J. *Biomater. Sci., Polym. Ed.* 2011, 22,893.
[210] Arias, J. L. *Molecules* 2008, 13, 2340.
[211] Barry, S. E. *Int. J. Hyperthermia* 2008, 24, 451.
[212] Zavisová, V.; Koneracká, M.; Štrbak, O.; Tomasovicová, N.;Kopcanský, P.; Timko, M.; Vavra, I. J. *Magn. Magn. Mater.* 2007, 311, 379.
[213] Weissleder, R.; Tung, C. H.; Mahmood, U.; Bogdanov, A., Jr.Nat. *Biotechnol.* 1999, 17, 375.
[214] Tung, C. H.; Mahmood, U.; Bredow, S.; Weissleder, R. *Cancer Res.* 2000, 60, 4953.
[215] Lübbe, A. S.; Bergemann, C.; Brock, J.; McClure, D. G. J. *Magn. Magn. Mater.* 1999, 194, 149.
[216] Grief, A. D.; Richardson, G. J. *Magn. Magn. Mater.* 2005, 293,455.
[217] Scott, G.; Peterson, C.; Hohn, C.; Bittner, C. J. *Magn. Magn.Mater.* 1999, 194, 132.
[218] Pankhurst, Q. A.; Connolly, J.; Jones, S. K.; Dobson, J. J. *Phys. D: Appl. Phys.* 2003, 36, R167.
[219] Chen, H. T.; Ebner, A. D.; Rosengart, A. J.; Kaminski, M. D.;Ritter, J. A. J. *Magn. Magn. Mater.* 2004, 284, 181.
[220] Avilés, M. O.; Ebner, A. D.; Ritter, J. A. J. *Magn. Magn. Mater.*2008, 320, 2640.
[221] Gang, J.; Park, S. B.; Hyung, W.; Choi, E. H.; Wen, J.; Kim, H.S.; Shul, Y. G.; Haam, S.; Song, S. Y. J. *Drug Targeting* 2007, 15, 445.
[222] Lübbe, A. S.; Bergemann, C.; Riess, H.; Schriever, F.;Reichardt, P.; Possinger, K.; Matthias, M.; Dörken, B.; Herrmann,F.; Gürtler, R.; Hohenberger, P.; Haas, N.; Sohr, R.; Sander, B.;Lemke, A. J.; Ohlendorf, D.; Huhnt, W.; Huhn, D. *Cancer Res.* 1996,56, 4686.
[223] Yu, M. K.; Jeong, Y. Y.; Park, J.; Park, S.; Kim, J. W.; Min, J. J.;Kim, K.; Jon, S. *Angew. Chem., Int. Ed.* 2008, 47, 5362.
[224] Zhang, J. Q.; Zhang, Z. R.; Yang, H.; Tan, Q. Y.; Qin, S. R.;Qiu, X. L. *Pharm. Res.* 2005, 22, 573.
[225] Fortin-Ripoche, J. P.; Martina, M. S.; Gazeau, F.; Menager, C.;Wilhelm, C.; Bacri, J. C.; Lesieur, S.; Clement, O. *Nanomedicine* 2010,5, 1173.
[226] Gultepe, E.; Reynoso, F. J.; Jhaveri, A.; Kulkarni, P.; Nagesha,D.; Ferris, C.; Harisinghani, M.; Campbell, R. B.; Sridhar, S. *Nanomedicine* (London) 2010, 5, 1173.
[227] Torchilin, P. *Nat. Rev. Drug Discovery* 2005, 4, 145.

[228] Virooonchatapan, E.; Sato, H.; Ueno, M.; Adachi, I.; Tazawa, K.;Horikoshi, I. *Life Sci.* 1996, 58, 2251.

[229] Lübbe, A. S.; Alexiou, C.; Bergemann, C. J. *Surg. Res.* 2001, 95,200.

[230] Peer, D.; Karp, J. M.; Hong, S.; Farokhzad, O. C.; Margalit, R.; Langer, R. *Nat. Nanotechnol.* 2007, 2, 751.

[231] Holgado, M. A.; Martín-Banderas, L.; Álvarez-Fuentes, J.; Fernández-Arévalo, M.; Arias, J. L. *Curr. Med. Chem.* 2012, 19, 3188.

[232] Clares, B.; Ruiz, M. A.; Gallardo, V.; Arias, J. L. *Curr. Med.Chem.* 2012, 19, 3203.

[233] Varner, J. A.; Cheresh, D. A. *Curr. Opin. Cell Biol.* 1996, 8, 724.

[234] Vandewalle, B.; Granier, A. M.; Peyrat, J. P.; Bonneterre, J.;Lefebvre, J. *J. Cancer Res. Clin. Oncol.* 1985, 110, 71.

[235] Farokhzad, O. C.; Jon, S.; Khademhosseini, A.; Tran, T. N.;Lavan, D. A.; Langer, R. *Cancer Res.* 2004, 64, 7668.

[236] Herr, J. K.; Smith, J. E.; Medley, C. D.; Shangguan, D.; Tan, W. *Anal. Chem.* 2006, 78, 2918.

[237] Smith, J. E.; Medley, C. D.; Tang, Z.; Shangguan, D.; Lofton,C.; Tan, W. *Anal. Chem.* 2007, 79, 3075.

[238] Yigit, M. V.; Mazumdar, D.; Kim, H. K.; Lee, J. H.; Odintsov,B.; Lu, Y. *Chem Bio Chem* 2007, 8, 1675.

[239] Yigit, M. V.; Mazumdar, D.; Lu, Y. *Bioconjugate Chem.* 2008,19, 412.

[240] Cerdan, S.; Lotscher, H. R.; Kunnecke, B.; Seelig, J. *Magn.Reson. Med.* 1989, 12, 151.

[241] Weissleder, R.; Lee, A. S.; Fischman, A. J.; Reimer, P.; Shen, T.;Wilkinson, R.; Callahan, R. J.; Brady, T. J. *Radiology* 1991, 181, 245.

[242] Tiefenauer, L. X.; Kuhne, G.; Andres, R. Y. *Bioconjugate Chem.*1993, 4, 347.

[243] Artemov, D.; Mori, N.; Okollie, B.; Bhujwala, Z. M. *Magn.Reson. Med.* 2003, 49, 403.

[244] Artemov, D.; Mori, N.; Ravi, R.; Bhujwalla, Z. M. *Cancer Res.*2003, 63, 2723.

[245] Huh, Y. M.; Jun, Y. W.; Song, H. T.; Kim, S.; Choi, J. S.; Lee, J.H.; Yoon, S.; Kim, K. S.; Shin, J. S.; Suh, J. S.; Cheon, J. J. *Am. Chem.Soc.* 2005, 127, 12387.

[246] Foon, K. A. *Cancer Res.* 1989, 49, 1621.

[247] Arias, J. L. *Expert Opin. Drug Delivery* 2011, 8, 1589.

[248] Kohler, N.; Sun, C.; Fichtenholtz, A.; Gunn, J.; Fang, C.;Zhang, M. Q. *Small* 2006, 2, 785.

[249] Santra, S.; Kaittanis, C.; Grimm, J.; Perez, J. M. *Small* 2009, 5,1862.

[250] Maeng, J. H.; Lee, D. H.; Jung, K. H.; Bae, Y. H.; Park, I. S.;Jeong, S.; Jeon, Y. S.; Shim, C. K.; Kim, W.; Kim, J.; Lee, J.; Lee, Y. M.;Kim, J. H.; Kim, W. H.; Hong, S. S. *Biomaterials* 2010, 31, 4995.

[251] Arias, J. L.; Reddy, L. H.; Othman, M.; Gillet, B.; Desmaële, D.;Zouhiri, F.; Dosio, F.; Gref, R.; Couvreur, P. *ACS Nano* 2011, 5, 1513.

[252] Rowe, M. D.; Thamm, D. H.; Kraft, S. L.; Boyes, S. G. *Biomacromolecules* 2009, 10, 983.

[253] Bagalkot, V.; Zhang, L.; Levy-Nissenbaum, E.; Jon, S.; Kantoff,P. W.; Langer, R.; Farokhzad, O. C. *Nano Lett.* 2007, 7, 3065.

[254] Kim, J.; Kim, H. S.; Lee, N.; Kim, T.; Kim, H.; Yu, T.; Song, I.C.; Moon, W. K.; Hyeon, T. *Angew. Chem., Int.* Ed. 2008, 47, 8438.

[255] Camilleri-Broet, S.; Hardy-Bessard, A. C.; Le Tourneau, A.;Paraiso, D.; Levrel, O.; Leduc, B.; Bain, S.; Orfeuvre, H.; Audouin, J.;Pujade-Lauraine, E. *Ann. Oncol.* 2004, 15, 104.

[256] Tovey, S. M.; Brown, S.; Doughty, J. C.; Mallon, E. A.; Cooke,T. G.; Edwards, J. *Br. J. Cancer* 2009, 100, 680.

[257] Yang, J.; Lee, C. H.; Ko, H. J.; Suh, J. S.; Yoon, H. G.; Lee, K.;Huh, Y. M.; Haam, S. *Angew. Chem., Int. Ed.* 2007, 46, 8836.

[258] Schmieder, A. H.; Caruthers, S. D.; Zhang, H.; Williams, T. A.;Robertson, J. D.; Wickline, S. A.; Lanza, G. M. *FASEB J.* 2008, 22,4179.

[259] Alexiou, C.; Arnold, W.; Klein, R.; Parak, F. G.; Hulin, P.; Bergemann, C.; Erhardt, W.; Wagenpfeil, S.; Lübbe, A. S. *Cancer Res.* 2000, 60, 6641.

[260] Chertok, B.; David, A. E.; Yang, V. C. *Biomaterials* 2010, 31,6317.

[261] Poore, G. A.; Senyei, A. E. *Eur. J. Cancer Clin. Oncol.* 1983, 19,141.

[262] Gorby, Y. A.; Beveridge, T. J.; Blakemore, R. P. *J. Bacteriol.*1988, 170, 834.

[263] Grünberg, K.; Müller, E. C.; Otto, A.; Reszka, R.; Linder, D.;Kube, M.; Reinhardt, R.; Schüler, D. *Appl. Environ. Microbiol.* 2004, 70,1040.

[264] Matsunaga, T.; Maeda, Y.; Yoshino, T.; Takeyama, H.;Takahashi, M.; Ginya, H.; Aasahina, J.; Tajima, H. *Anal. Chim. Acta* 2007, 597, 331.

[265] Takeyama, H.; Yamazawa, A.; Nakamura, C.; Matsunaga, T. *Biotechnol. Tech.* 1995, 9, 355.

[266] Sun, J. B.; Duan, J. H.; Dai, S. L.; Ren, J.; Zhang, Y. D.; Tian, J.S.; Li, Y. *Cancer Lett.* 2007, 258, 109.

[267] Chen, H.; Langer, R. *Pharm. Res.* 1997, 14, 537.

[268] Zhang, J.; Misra, R. D. *Acta Biomater.* 2007, 3, 838.

[269] Yuan, Q.; Venkatasubramanian, R.; Hein, S.; Misra, R. D. *Acta Biomater.* 2008, 4, 1024.

[270] Willmott, N. *Cancer Treat. Rev.* 1987, 14, 143.

[271] Ma, Y. H.; Hsu, Y. W.; Chang, Y. J.; Hua, M. Y.; Chen, J. P.;Wu, T. J. Magn. *Magn. Mater.* 2007, 311, 342.

[272] Torchilin, V. P.; Paptov, M. I.; Orekova, N. M.; Belyaev, A. A.;Petrov, A. D.; Ragimov, S. E. *Haemostasis* 1988, 18, 113.

[273] Larsen, C.; Østergaard, J.; Larsen, S. W.; Jensen, H.; Jacobsen,S.; Lindegaard, C.; Andersen, P. H. J. *Pharm. Sci.* 2008, 97, 4622.

[274] Dhalla, N. S.; Temsah, R. M.; Netticadan, T. J. *Hypertension* 2000, 18, 655.

[275] Chorny, M.; Hood, E.; Levy, R. J.; Muzykantov, V. R. J. *Controlled Release* 2010, 146, 144.

[276] Kopke, R. D.; Wassel, R. A.; Mondalek, F.; Grady, B.; Chen,K.; Liu, J.; Gibson, D.; Dormer, K. J. *Audiol. Neurotol.* 2006, 11, 123.

[277] Forbes, Z. G.; Yellen, B. B.; Halverson, D. S.; Fridman, G.;Barbee, K. A.; Friedman, G. *IEEE Trans. Biomed. Eng.* 2008, 55, 643.

[278] Goldberg, S. L.; Loussararian, A.; De Gregorio, J.; Di Mario,C.; Albiero, R.; Colombo, A. J. *Am. Coll. Cardiol.* 2001, 37, 1019.

[279] McDowell, G.; Slevin, M.; Krupinski, J. Vasc. Cell. 2011, 3, 8.

[280] Kempe, H.; Kempe, M. *Biomaterials* 2010, 31, 9499.

[281] Chorny, M.; Fishbein, I.; Yellen, B. B.; Alferiev, I. S.; Bakay, M.;Ganta, S.; Adamo, R.; Amiji, M.; Friedman, G.; Levy, R. J. *Proc. Natl.Acad. Sci. USA*. 2010, 107, 8346.

[282] Natarajan, A.; Xiong, C. Y.; Gruettner, C.; DeNardo, G. L.; DeNardo, S. *J. Cancer Biother. Radiopharm*. 2008, 23, 82.

[283] Chen, J.; Wu, H.; Han, D.; Xie, C. *Cancer Lett.* 2006, 231, 169.

[284] Natarajan, A.; Gruettner, C.; Ivkov, R.; DeNardo, G. L.; Mirick,G.; Yuan, A.; Foreman, A.; DeNardo, S. J. *Bioconjugate Chem.* 2008,19, 1211.

[285] Konan, Y. N.; Gurny, R.; Allemann, E. J. *Photochem. Photobiol.* B 2002, 66, 89.

[286] Park, S. I.; Hwang, Y. H.; Lim, J. H.; Kim, J. H.; Yun, H. I.;Kim, C. O. *J. Magn. Magn. Mater.* 2006, 304, e403.

[287] Primo, F. L.; Macaroff, P. P.; Lacava, Z. G. M.; Azevedo, R. B.;Morais, P. C.; Tedesco, A. C. J. *Magn. Magn. Mater.* 2007, 310, 2838.

[288] Primo, F. L.; Michieleto, L.; Rodrigues, M. A. M.; Macaroff, P.P.; Morais, P. C.; Lacava, Z. G. M.; Bentley, M. V. L. B.; Tedesco, A. C.J. *Magn. Magn. Mater.* 2007, 311, 354.

[289] Huang, P.; Li, Z.; Lin, J.; Yang, D.; Gao, G.; Xu, C.; Bao, L.;Zhang, C.; Wang, K.; Song, H.; Hu, H.; Cui, D. *Biomaterials* 2011, 32,3447.
[290] Lai, C. W.; Wang, Y. H.; Lai, C. H.; Yang, M. J.; Chen, C. Y.;Chou, P. T.; Chan, C. S.; Chi, Y.; Chen, Y. C.; Hsiao, J. K. *Small* 2008,4, 218.
[291] Jordan, A.; Scholz, R.; Wust, P.; Fähling, H.; Felix, R. J. *Magn.Magn. Mater.* 1999, 201, 413.
[292] Ito, A.; Tanaka, K.; Honda, H.; Abe, S.; Yamaguchi, H.; Kobayashi, T. J. *Biosci. Bioeng.* 2003, 96, 364.
[293] Ito, A.; Shinkai, M.; Honda, H.; Kobayashi, T. J. *Biosci. Bioeng.*2005, 100, 1.
[294] Hilger, I.; Hergt, R.; Kaiser, W. A. J. *Magn. Magn. Mater.* 2005,293, 314.
[295] Campbell, R. B. *Nanomedicine* (London) 2007, 2, 649.
[296] Jordan, A.; Scholz, R.; Maier-Hauff, K.; Johannsen, M.; Wust,P.; Nadobny, J.; Schirra, H.; Schmidt, H.; Deger, S.; Loening, S.;Lanksch, W.; Felix, R. J. *Magn. Magn. Mater.* 2001, 225, 118.
[297] Moroz, P.; Jones, S. K.; Gray, B. N. *Int. J. Hyperthermia* 2002,18, 267.
[298] Tanaka, K.; Ito, A.; Kobayashi, T.; Kawamura, T.; Shimada, S.;Matsumoto, K.; Saida, T.; Honda, H. J. *Biosci. Bioeng.* 2005, 100, 112.
[299] Glöckl, G.; Hergt, R.; Zeisberger, M.; Dutz, S.; Nagel, S.; Weitschies, W. *J. Phys. Cond. Matter.* 2006, 18, S2935.
[300] Huber, D. L. Small 2005, 1, 482.
[301] Hilger, I.; Andrä, W.; Hergt, R.; Hiergeist, R.; Schubert, H.;Kaiser, W. A. *Radiology* 2001, 218, 570.
[302] Jordan, A.; Scholz, R.; Maier-Hauff, K.; van Landeghem, F. K.H.; Waldoefner, N.; Teichgraeber, U.; Pinkernelle, J.; Bruhn, H.;Neumann, F.; Thiesen, B.; von Deimling, A.; Felix, R. *J. Neuroonco*l.2006, 78, 7.
[303] Yan, S.; Zhang, D.; Gu, N.; Zheng, J.; Ding, A.; Wang, Z.; Xing,B.; Ma, M.; Zhang, Y. *J. Nanosci. Nanotechnol.* 2005, 5, 1185.
[304] Babincov, M.; Altanerov, V.; Altaner, C.; Bergemann, C.;Babinec, P. *IEEE Trans. Nanobiosci.* 2008, 7, 15.
[305] Ang, K. L.; Venkatraman, S.; Ramanujan, R. V. Mater. *Sci. Eng.,C* 2007, 27, 347.
[306] Lehmann, J.; Natarajan, A.; Denardo, G. L.; Ivkov, R.;Foreman, A. R.; Catapano, C.; Mirick, G.; Ouang, T.; Gruettner, C.; Denardo, S. J. *Cancer Biother. Radiopharm.* 2008, 23, 265.
[307] Hilger, I.; Hiergeist, R.; Hergt, R.; Winnefeld, K.; Schubert, H.;Kaiser, W. A. *Invest. Radiol.* 2002, 37, 580.

[308] Yukumi, S.; Watanabe, Y.; Horiuchi, A.; Doi, T.; Sato, K.;Yoshida, M.; Machara, T.; Aono, H.; Naohara, T.; Kawachi, K. *Anticancer Res*. 2008, 28, 69.

[309] Kong, G.; Braun, R. D.; Dewhirst, M. W. *Cancer Res*. 2000, 60,4440.

[310] Needham, D.; Anyarambhatla, G.; Kong, G.; Dewhirst, M. W. *Cancer Res*. 2000, 60, 1197.

[311] Tashjian, J. A.; Dewhirst, M. W.; Needham, D.; Viglianti, B. L. *Int. J. Hyperthermia* 2008, 24, 79.

[312] Karino, T.; Koga, S.; Maeta, M. *Surg. Today* 1988, 18, 276.

[313] Horsman, M. R.; Overgaard, J. *Int. J. Hyperthermia* 1997, 13,141.

[314] Kong, G.; Dewhirst, M. W. *Int. J. Hyperthermia* 1999, 15, 345.

[315] Cope, D.; Dewhirst, M.; Friedman, H.; Bigner, D.; Zalutsky, M. *Cancer Res.* 1990, 50, 1803.

[316] Hosono, M. N.; Hosono, M.; Endo, K.; Ueda, R.; Onoyama, Y.J. Nucl. Med. 1994, 35, 504.Johannsen, M.; Gneveckow, U.; Eckelt, L.; Feussner, A.;Waldöfner, N.; Scholz, R.; Deger, S.; Wust, P.; Loening, S. A.; Jordan,A. *Int. J. Hyperthermia* 2005, 21, 637.

[317] Johannsen, M.; Gneveckow, U.; Taymoorian, K.; Thiesen, B.;Waldöfner, N.; Scholz, R.; Jung, K.; Jordan, A.; Wust, P.; Loening, S. A. *Int. J. Hyperthermia* 2007, 23, 315.

[318] Johannsen, M.; Gneveckow, U.; Thiesen, B.; Taymoorian, K.;Cho, C. H.; Waldöfner, N.; Scholz, R.; Jordan, A.; Loening, S. A.;Wust, P. *Eur. Urol.* 2007, 52, 1653.

[319] Wust, P.; Gneveckow, U.; Johannsen, M.; Böhmer, D.; Henkel,T.; Kahmann, F.; Sehouli, J.; Felix, R.; Ricke, J.; Jordan, A. *Int. J. Hyperthermia* 2006, 22, 673.

[320] Maier-Hauff, K.; Rothe, R.; Scholz, R.; Gneveckow, U.; Wust,P.; Thiesen, B.; Feussner, A.; Deimling, A.; Waldoefner, N.; Felix, R.;Jordan, A. *J. Neurooncol*. 2007, 81, 53.

[321] Müller, S. Nanomed. *Nanotechnol. Biol. Med*. 2009, 5, 387.

[322] Kroft, L. J. M.; Doornbos, J.; van der Geest, R. J.; van derLaarse, A.; van der Meulen, H.; de Roos, A. *Magn. Reson. Imaging* 1998, 16, 755.

[323] Terreno, E.; Castelli, D. D.; Viale, A.; Aime, S. *Chem. Rev*. 2010, 110, 3019.

[324] Vogl, T. J.; Hammerstingl, R.; Schwarz, W.; Mack, M. G.; Muller, P. K.; Pegios, W.; Keck, H.; Eibl-Eibesfeldt, V.; Hoelzl, J.;Woessmer, B.; Bergman, V.; Felix, R. *Radiology* 1996, 198, 881.

[325] Oswald, P.; Clement, O.; Chambon, C.; Schouman-Claeys, E.;Frija, G. *Magn. Reson. Imaging* 1997, 15, 1025.

[326] Shamsi, K.; Balzer, T.; Saini, S.; Ros, P. R.; Nelson, R. C.;Carter, E. C.; Tollerfield, S.; Niendorf, H. P. *Radiology* 1998, 206, 365.

[327] Abe, Y.; Yamashita, Y.; Namimoto, T.; Tang, Y.; Takahashi, M. *Radiat. Med.* 2000, 18, 97.

[328] Reimer, P.; Tombach, B. *Eur. Radiol.* 1998, 8, 1198.

[329] Reddy, L. H.; Couvreur, P. *J. Hepatol.* 2011, 55, 1461.

[330] Lind, K.; Kresse, M.; Debus, N. P.; Müller, R. H. J. *Drug Target.*2002, 10, 221.

[331] Mack, M. G.; Balzer, J. O.; Straub, R.; Eichler, V.; Vogl, T. *J. Radiology* 2002, 222, 239.

[332] Thorek, D. L. J.; Chen, A. K.; Czupryna, J.; Tsourkas, A. *Ann. Biomed.* Eng. 2006, 34, 23.

[333] Guimaraes, R.; Clément, O.; Bittoun, J.; Carnot, F.; Frija, G. *Am. J. Roentgenol.* 1994, 162, 201.

[334] Harisinghani, M. G.; Saksena, M. A.; Hahn, P. F.; King, B.;Kim, J.; Torabi, M. T.; Weissleder, R. *Am. J. Roentgenol.* 2006, 186,144.

[335] Islam, T.; Harisinghani, M. G. *Cancer Biomarkers* 2009, 5, 61.

[336] Anzai, Y.; Piccoli, C. W.; Outwater, E. K.; Stanford, W.;Bluemke, D. A.; Nurenberg, P.; Saini, S.; Maravilla, K. R.; Feldman, D.E.; Schmiedl, U. P.; Brunberg, J. A.; Francis, I. R.; Harms, S. E.; Som,P. M.; Tempany, C. M. *Radiology* 2003, 228, 777.

[337] Will, O.; Purkayastha, S.; Chan, C.; Athanasiou, T.; Darzi, A.W.; Gedrovc, W.; Tekkis, P. P. *Lancet Oncol.* 2006, 7, 52.

[338] Dousset, V.; Delalande, C.; Ballarino, L.; Quesson, B.; Seilhan,D.; Coussemacq, M.; Thiaudiére, D.; Brochet, B.; Canioni, P.; Caillé, J.M. *Magn. Reson. Med.* 1999, 41, 329.

[339] Müller, R. N.; Gillis, P.; Moiny, F.; Roch, A. *Magn. Reson. Med.*1991, 22, 178.

[340] Chambon, C.; Clement, O.; Le Blanche, A.; Schouman-Claeys, E.; Frija, G. *Magn. Reson. Imaging* 1993, 11, 509.

[341] Schmitz, S. A.; Coupland, S. E.; Gust, R.; Winterhalter, S.;Wagner, S.; Kresse, M.; Semmler, W.; Wolf, K. *J. Invest. Radiol.* 2000,35, 460.

[342] Ruehm, S. G.; Corot, C.; Vogt, P.; Kolb, S.; Debatin, J. F. *Circulation* 2001, 103, 415.

[343] Trivedi, R. A.; Mallawarachi, C.; U-King-Im, J. M.; Graves, M.J.; Horsley, J.; Goddard, M. J.; Brown, A.; Wang, L.; Kirkpatrick, P. J.;Brown, J.; Gillard, J. H. *Arterioscler. Thromb. Vasc. Biol.* 2006, 26, 1601.

[344] Virmani, R.; Kolodgie, F. D.; Burke, A. P.; Finn, A. V.; Gold, H.K.; Tulenko, T. N.; Wrenn, S. P.; Narula, J. Arterioscler., *Thromb., Vasc.Biol.* 2005, 25, 2054.

[345] Kooi, M. E.; Cappendijk, V. C.; Cleutjens, K.; Kessels, A. G.H.; Kitslaar, P.; Borgers, M.; Frederik, P. M; Daemen, M.; vanEngelshoven, J. M. A. *Circulation* 2003, 107, 2453.

[346] Rausch, M.; Sauter, A.; Fröhlich, J.; Neubacher, U.; Radü, E.W.; Rudin, M. *Magn. Reson. Med.* 2001, 46, 1018.

[347] Saleh, A.; Schroeter, M.; Jonkmanns, C.; Hartung, H. P.;MoE dder, U.; Jander, S. *Brain* 2004, 127, 1670.

[348] Neuwelt, E. A.; Varallyay, P.; Bago, A. G.; Muldoon, L. L.;Nesbit, G.; Nixon, R. Neuropathol. *Appl. Neurobiol.* 2004, 30, 456.

[349] Hunt, M. A.; Bago, A. G.; Neuwelt, E. A. *Am. J. Neuroradiol.*2005, 26, 1084.

[350] Baeten, K.; Hendriks, J. J.; Hellings, N.; Theunissen, E.;Vanderlocht, J.; Ryck, L. D.; Gelan, J.; Stinissen, P.; Adriaensens, P. *Neuroimmunol.* 2008, 195, 1.

[351] Dousset, V.; Brochet, B.; Deloire, M. S.; Lagoarde, L.; Barroso,B.; Caille, J. M.; Petry, K. G. *Am. J. Neuroradiol.* 2006, 27, 1000.

[352] Zhang, Y.; Dodd, S. J.; Hendrich, K. S.; Williams, M.; Ho, C. *Kidney Int.* 2000, 58, 1300.

[353] Kanno, C.; Lee, P. C.; Dodd, S. J.; Williams, M.; Griffith, B. P.;Ho, C. J. *Thorac. Cardiovasc. Surg.* 2000, 120, 923.

[354] Bierry, G.; Jehl, F.; Neuville, A.; Lefevre, S.; Robert, P.;Kremer, S.; Dietemann, J. L. *Am. J. Roentgenol.* 2010, 194, W521.

[355] Lutz, A. M.; Seemayer, C.; Corot, C.; Gay, R. E.; Goepfert, K.;Michel, B. A.; Marincek, B.; Gay, S.; Weishaupt, D. *Radiology* 2004,233, 149.

[356] Kanno, S.; Wu, Y. J.; Lee, P. C.; Dodd, S. J.; Williams, M.;Griffith, B. P.; Ho, C. *Circulation* 2001, 104, 934.

[357] Sosnovik, D. E.; Nahrendorf, M.; Weissleder, R. *Circulation* 2007, 115, 2076.

[358] Sosnovik, D. E.; Nahrendorf, M.; Deliolanis, N.; Novikov, M.;Aikawa, E.; Josephson, L.; Rosenzweig, A.; Weissleder, R.; Ntziachristos, V. *Circulation* 2007, 115, 1384.

[359] Sosnovik, D. E.; Nahrendorf, M.; Weissleder, R. Basic Res.Cardiol. 2008, 103, 122.

[360] Kubinova, S.; Sykova, E. Minim. *Invasive Ther. Allied Technol.* 2010, 19, 144.

[361] Ito, A.; Takizawa, Y.; Honda, H.; Hata, K.; Kagami, H.; Ueda,M.; Kobayashi, T. *Tissue Eng*. 2004, 10, 833.

[362] Shimuzu, K.; Ito, A.; Honda, H. J. Biomed. Mater. Res., *Part B: Appl. Biomater*. 2006, 77B, 265.

[363] Sasaki, T.; Iwasaki, N.; Kohno, K.; Kishimoto, M.; Majima, T.;Nishimura, S. I.; Minami, A. J. *Biomed. Mater. Res*. 2008, 86A, 969.

[364] Ito, A.; Akiyama, H.; Kawabe, Y.; Kamihira, M. *J. Biosci. Bioeng*. 2007, 104, 288.

[365] Ito, A.; Ino, K.; Hayashida, M.; Kobayashi, T.; Matsunuma, H.;Kagami, H.; Ueda, M.; Honda, H. *Tissue Eng*. 2005, 11, 1553.

[366] Shimuzu, K.; Ito, A.; Arinobe, M.; Murase, Y.; Iwata, Y.; Narita,Y.; Kagami, H.; Ueda, M.; Honda, H. J. *Biosci. Bioeng*. 2007, 103, 472.

[367] Shimuzu, K.; Ito, A.; Yoshida, T.; Yamada, Y.; Ueda, M.;Honda, H. J. Biomed. Mater. Res., *Part B: Appl. Biomater*. 2007, 82B,471.

[368] Shimuzu, K.; Ito, A.; Honda, H. J. *Biosci. Bioeng*. 2007, 104,171.

[369] Oshima, S.; Ishikawa, M.; Mochizuki, Y.; Kobayashi, T.;Yasunaga, Y.; Ochi, M. J. *Bone Joint Surg*. Br. 2010, 92, 1606.

[370] Kobayashi, T.; Ochi, M.; Yanada, S.; Ishikawa, M.; Adachi, N.;Deie, M.; Arihiro, K. *Arthroscopy* 2008, 24, 69.

[371] Shimuzu, K.; Ito, A.; Yoshida, T.; Miwa, K.; Ishiguro, H.;Numaguchi, Y.; Murohara, T.; Kodama, I.; Honda, H. *Biotechnol.Bioeng*. 2007, 96, 803.

In: *In Vivo* Imaging: New Research
Editors: R. Hough and J. Camarillo
ISBN: 978-1-62948-633-8

Chapter 3

In Vivo Imaging of Bone

***Liam Lawlor*[1], *Ronald Grigg*[2] *and Xuebin Yang*[1,*]**
[1]Biomaterials and Tissue Engineering Group,
School of Dentistry, University of Leeds, UK
[2]The MIDAS Centre, School of Chemistry,
University of Leeds, UK

Abstract

Bone is a specialised connective tissue comprising of cells and bone matrix. The two main constituents of bone are an inorganic mineralised component and a highly organised collagen organic component. It responds to stimuli such as mechanical forces, hormone levels and disease [1]. Unlike the other connective tissues, the extracellular matrix of bone is mineralised, making it a hard, unyielding substance ideally suited for its supportive and protective functions. Depending on the location, different types of bone are different in structure and shape, which can be apparent when bone is imaged.

Non-invasive *in vivo* imaging of bone can be a useful tool for the diagnosis and assessment of bone quality, allowing the monitoring of the bone in real time during physiological/pathological events such as fractures, disease, healing and remodelling. Discovered over 100 years ago, the most commonly used method for bone imaging is still X-ray spectroscopy [2]. Since then, many new techniques have been developed.

* E-mail: X.B.Yang@leeds.ac.uk.

For *in vivo* work, this will increase the quality of the outcome (via self-comparative studies) and reduce the number of animals required, with advantageous economic and ethical implications.

This chapter provides an overview of techniques for *in vivo* bone imaging, including the better established methods of X-ray [3], micro computed tomography [4], magnetic resonance imaging [5], SPECT/PET nuclear imaging technologies [6] and ultrasound [7]. It also covers some more modern and less prevalent methods, such as fluorescence [8] and bioluminescent [9]. The advantages, limitations and indications of the application of each technique are also discussed.

Introduction

There is a highlighted clinical need for the imaging of bone and related tissue. In particular, age-related and osteoporotic related fractures are a worldwide major health problem. Furthermore, bone fractures and bone loss as a result of traumatic injuries, congenital deformities and pathological degenerations result in millions of people every year requiring some form of medical intervention to deal with bone related health issues [10, 11].

To tackle these clinical challenges animal models have become an integral part of research at both a university and an industrial level. Animal models are an essential step in translational research, integral to taking clinical therapies from research hypothesis to phase three clinical trials. The results of research conducted *in vitro* needs to be confirmed *in vivo* [12].

Animal models have been widely used in such cases as drug screening processes (where bone densities often have to be monitored) [13], fracture healing [14], bone metabolic diseases [15], bone genetic disorders [9], cancer research [16] and bone tissue regeneration/engineering studies [12, 15, 17]. Since these are dynamic procedures, it is often essential to monitor how the bones of animals are being affected during these studies, and non-invasive *in vivo* imaging is a useful tool for the diagnosis and assessment of bone quality.

Invasive methods involve either taking biopsies or terminating animals at set time points, which requires a large number of animals, and also makes self-comparison studies, where the animal acts as its own control, impossible. In contrast, non-invasive imaging allows the monitoring of bone in real time, during physiological and pathological events such as bone fracture, disease, healing and remodelling. Advances in *in vivo* imaging allow the non-invasive study of a single subject, a self-comparison study, which greatly improves the quality of the outcome of *in vivo* studies. These studies also have the added benefit of reducing the number of animals required for studies, with both economic and ethical advantages.

The first imaging of bone was by accident in 1895, when Wilhelm Röntgen created an X-ray image of his hand. This was the beginning of modern medical imaging, which has led researchers to a number of options today for *in vivo* imaging of bone [18]. After over one hundred years, X-ray is still a conventional imaging technology in clinical practice for bone and joints, although there are limitations to the technology. To overcome these deficits, other techniques, such as CT, MRI, fluorescence and ultrasound imaging have been developed. However, each of these methods has its own advantages and limitations. The choice of method for *in vivo* imaging of bone will depend on the tissues and organs to be imaged, their location, physiological/pathological conditions and the time periods over which the imaging is required. Thus, understanding the tissue's structure and potential alterations, such as when diseased, is important.

Bone Biology and Structure

Bone is often crudely thought of simply as a rigid mass of hard, connective tissue which, with cartilage, makes up the skeletal system. However, it is actually a living organ and consists of cells and bone matrix with a specific dynamic structure ideally suited for its supportive, protective and movement (in conjunction with cartilage) functions in the skeleton [19]. Being highly inorganic, bone can also have a homeostatic role, acting as a reservoir for minerals and ions, as well as playing a role in blood regulation [20]. Because bone is in a dynamic state, it is constantly being renewed and reconstructed throughout the lifetime of an individual.

Bone as an organ, can be classified according to its shape, gross appearance and developmental origin. Bone size, shape, structure and strength can vary drastically across different species, sexes, races, with different genetic makeups or with age. The structure can be very complex and vary depending on its location and function. Traditionally, cortical bone (also known as compact bone) and trabecular bone (also known as cancellous or spongy bone) are the two key types of the bone which are referred to in text books and publications [21]. Cortical and trabecular bone are macroscopic classifications of bone, at the microscopic level bone is classified as woven or lamellar bone [22]. The physical properties of bone mostly depend on the anatomical site of the bone (the location) and the age and history (medical and lifestyle) of the individual.

Cortical bone can be characterised by two distinct collagen fibre structures: either running in a single direction, parallel to each other (lamellae) or concentrically organized around a vascular canal, called Haversian systems or osteons [10, 23]. Each canal is lined with an endosteum, a thin layer of connective tissue, and contains blood vessels, nerves and loose connective tissue [19]. These vascularised Haversian canals provide an essential blood supply to the bone, necessary for nutrition and waste disposal. Cortical bone is mainly found on the outside of long bone structures, forming a shell [24].

In contrast to cortical bone, trabecular bone is found towards the centre of the cortical bone shells and in areas of the skeleton where bone experience compression, such as in cavities at the end of long bones. It consists of lamellae in an irregular lattice network without the presence of osteons [20, 24]. This conveys the trabecular bone elastic properties, which aid it in load bearing capacity.

In general, bone matrix consists of roughly 15-25% water, 30% organic substance and 70% inorganic material, but this is dependent on age and type of the bone tissue [22]. In adult mammals, about 90% of the organic matrix is type I collagen and minor constituents include bone sialoprotein (BSP), osteocalcin (OC), osteopontin (OP), osteonectin (ON), proteoglycans (PG) and glycoproteins (GP). The majority of the inorganic material in bone is hydroxyapatite, an inorganic mineral of calcium, phosphate and hydroxide [19, 22].

At a microscopic level, when new bone is being formed, such as in foetal formation, fracture sites and around some cancerous sites, the newly formed bone has an unorganised structure; it does not consist of highly organised collagen fibres. This new bone is known as woven bone and is relatively mechanically weak. It is typically replaced by lamellar bone in more mature bone, with an improved mechanical strength. Lamellar bone has a lower cell density and is well organised compare to woven immature bone [10, 22].

Bone is a direction dependent anisotropic material, which does not have a uniform or isotropic structure. This is because bone has grown to account for the loads applied to it. Cortical bone is stiffer and stronger when a force is applied in a longitudinal direction and it is stronger in compression than in tension. Trabecular bone is also anisotropic, with denser spongy bone found nearer the ends of joints. Bone has evolved to account for its function, so it can adequately cope with the everyday activities [24].

Bone marrow is located in the inner layer of bones and has many incredibly important functions, including producing red blood cells, fatty tissues and lymphocytes. Bone marrow is made of cell populations, notably bone marrow mesenchymal stem cells, different to other bone cell populations, which can vary drastically with the age of the bone and anatomical location. The cells in bone marrow are essential for tissue repair and regeneration, the maintenance of the immune system and for the formation of blood components [20].

Finally, except for the articulating ends, bone is covered by periosteum, a fibrous membrane. It contains osteoprogenitor cells which aid fracture healing and prevent bone formation from taking place outside of the bone [22].

Bone Formation

Bone is formed in one of two processes: intramembranous ossification or endochondral ossification. In intramembranous ossification, the bone matrix is secreted by osteoblasts onto a membrane. In endochondral ossification, the bone formation happens by deposition of bone onto a pre-formed cartilage matrix [25].

Bone remodelling is a coupled process of bone formation and bone resorption, undertaken by the joint effort of osteoblasts and osteoclasts, which together are known as the bone multicellular unit (BMU). Bone remodelling happens constantly throughout the whole life span of bone, in response to events such as fractures. In the process of bone remodelling osteoclasts remove bone from locations where there is less need for bone, to avoid unnecessary bulk, and osteoblasts form new bone where necessary. These processes take place to keep the skeleton in peak condition, as bone suffers constant stress and fatigue or other damage, such as from fractures. These processes are altered by a number of circumstances, including the age-related or disease changes which will be discussed later [19, 21].

The Clinical Need for the *In Vivo* Imaging of Bone

There are many factors which can influence bone remodelling. For example, the BMUs can be affected by age, the menopause in female subjects and a number of bone metabolic diseases and conditions. In patients suffering osteoporosis, the balance between bone formation and resorption is affected, resulting in a lifestyle affecting drop in bone density. The monitoring of bone densities is particularly important in high risk groups for osteoporosis, and is one of many examples of routine *in vivo* imaging [21].

Another incredibly prevalent disease which accounts for a large number of the studies involving the *in vivo* imaging of bone is arthritis [13, 26–29]. Osteoarthritis (OA) is the degradation and loss of hyaline cartilage and bone, resulting in pain and joint immobility [26]. Rheumatoid Arthritis (RA) is a chronic inflammatory disease of the joints which causes pain, swelling and eventually destruction of the joints [13].

Many different types of cancer can affect bone in one way or another. Not only cancers of the actual bone cells ("bone cancers"), but also other cancers in the body can cause bone metastases. These cancers can seed into bone, promoting osteoclast activity and resulting bone resorption. Being able to imaging these cancers and effects on bone non-invasively is an attractive prospect [1].

As well as the above mentioned bone affecting diseases and conditions, *in vivo* imaging of bone may also be utilised to monitor simple fractures and the healing process. Fracture response and healing is multi-step process, which begins with hematoma formation in the bone and surrounding tissue, immediately after fracture. The bone cells in the area can die, which can cause swelling in the region. The area then begins to be cleaned up by phagocytic cells. This is followed by fibrocartilaginous callus formation. At this stage, bone reconstruction is begun, with fibroblasts forming collagen fibres along with some cartilage matrix, formed by chondroblasts. After this process, osteoclasts and osteoblasts will work together to convert the fibrocartilaginous callus into a spongy bone callus - bone callus formation. This starts 3-4 weeks after the injury and continues until a firm bone structure is formed, after 2-3 months. The final step is remodelling, where excess matrix is removed, while compact bone is laid down to form a strong bone shaft. If the correct mechanical stimuli are applied, the bone will eventually have the same structure as the original bone. Clearly, at different stages of the fracture healing process, different imaging systems may be required to accurately monitor the bone healing and the quality of the bone formed [23].

To date, histology is still the "gold standard" when analysing tissues such as bone and it can provide a wealth of structural information of the bone. However, histology is an invasive technique, needing the acquisition of tissue, via biopsies or sacrifice of subjects. Thus, a number of different methods have been developed for non-invasive imaging of bone. These include the classical techniques X-ray, magnetic image resonance, computed tomography and ultrasound. Advances in non-invasive imaging technique attempt to match the accuracy of histology, and studies often use histology to validate their findings. X-ray imaging was the first of these techniques to be used in medical imaging.

X-ray

Introduction and History

X-rays were discovered in 1895 at University of Würzburg by Wilhelm Röntgen, for which he earned the Nobel Prize for Physics in 1901. After the initial discovery and their use as an entertainment tool, people quickly realised the usefulness of X-rays in bone imaging, and by World War I most hospitals had X-ray outfit. In the 1920s, a tool based on X-rays has also been developed for treating cancers. In the second half of the 20th century X-rays were integrated with computers, allowing their combination with other techniques and efficient image storage, leading to X-rays being cemented as a useful tool routinely used for the modern day *in vivo* imaging of bone [18]. In recent years more functional imaging utilising X-rays has improved and has led to exciting advances in *in vivo* imaging, it is not just a technique consigned to history [3]. Out of X-ray technology micro-CT technology was developed in the late 1960s, which will be outlined separately later.

Principles

Practically, X-rays are an electromagnetic wave which can interact with the object in question, producing a transmitted X-ray flux. This then generates a superimposed shadow based on the materials present. X-ray sensors detect the intensity of the X-rays as they propagate through the tissue and generate two dimensional (2D) images which highlight the changes in electron density between different materials and tissues. Materials such as bone, kidney stones and metal implants are shown in contrast to tissue [3, 30]. X-rays are electromagnetic waves which fall between 0.01 and 10 nanometers in length, with photon energies between 100 electron volts (eV) and 100 keV. Hard X-rays have photon energies above 10 keV (below 0.1 nm in wavelength) and soft X-rays account for the rest of the X-ray range [31].

Applications

The fundamentals of X-rays have changed very little since the 1895 discovery, and X-ray scanning has remained a relevant technology today. Since the early 20th century, X-rays have been widely used for non-invasive imaging of bone, metal implants and cavities in soft tissue, and as a tool for cancer treatments [3].

A key development of the X-ray technology was the invention of Dual-energy X-ray Absorptiometry (DEXA or DXA). It is widely used to measure body compositions of subjects and can give measurement of total-bone mineral density. The technology uses two X-ray beams of different energies to calculate of bone mineral density by subtracting the soft tissues out. DXA can be used for osteoporosis diagnosis and to monitor changes in bone density of subjects over time [32].

Advantages and Disadvantages

X-ray imaging has remained a relevant technology today because it is well understood, easily controllable and relatively cheap. Image generation is relatively quick and interpretation is simple, so structures such as fractured bone can be assessed. As with all imaging technologies, it is even more powerful when combined with other methods of generating data [33].

However, the 2D images generated by X-ray can sometimes be difficult to interpret with any great detail, due to the overlapping of structures not of interest, such as soft tissues. The inability to image these soft tissues is another major limitation of X-ray technology [3].

A major concern using X-ray technology is the associated ionising radiation. This can not only cause direct tissue reactions such as burns, but can also increase genomic instability of cells, leading to a high risk of causing cancers [34]. Thus, when undertaking *in vivo* studies, the doses of radiation animals receive should always be monitored and where possible minimised [35].

DXA can be used to high accuracy in animals used for *in vivo* studies such as mice [36] and chickens [37]. However the technology is limited when it comes to monitoring processes such as fractures and diseases such as osteoarthritis [32, 38]. Also, due to the fact that DXA is limited to only accurately being able to measure densities a maximum two materials with different absorptions, the studies on bone should be treated with caution. While DXA animal studies may match up to histological and other verification methods, the inaccuracies in human subjects are well understood. With bone marrow, fatty deposits and muscular tissue present, yet not being subtracted out from the readings, there are limitations to the technology [38].

Advances and Future Perspectives

To tackle the problem of soft tissue imaging, different contrast agents, such as Diatrizoate, have been introduced to enhance the imaging capability of X-ray for soft tissues. However these agents often have associated problems of toxicity, poor performance and high cost. Advances in the field ceased in the 1980s, until the potential of gold nanoparticles was realised in 2006. The injection of these agents was shown to improve X-ray contrast in soft tissues such as kidneys, blood vessels and tumours in mouse. The ability to image softer tissue around bone can still be useful in studies where not just bone needs to be imaged, with a single technology, such as X-ray [39]. Since bone is typically well imaged with X-ray technology, contrast agent development typically focuses on other, soft tissue, structures [3].

To overcome the issue of overlapping of soft tissue causing poor X-ray resolution, the technology was developed to be able to generate Three-Dimensional (3D) images of the targeted tissues. 3D scanners were used to acquire spatial distributions of tissues [3]. 3D Computed Tomography (CT) technology has surpassed X-ray technology for most instances of *in vivo* imaging of bone, because of the small size of subjects and the increased resolution available with micro-CT. Most studies today use micro-CT to assess bone and relevant structures *in vivo*.

Computed Tomography (CT)

Introduction and History

A major advance in the field of *in vivo* imaging of bone was the creation of the first X-ray Computed Tomography (CT) scanner in 1967. This was developed by Godfrey Hounsfield, who, along with Allan Cormack, was awarded a Nobel Prize in physiology and medicine for this in 1979.

In the early 1980s CT technology was further developed with the invention of the micro-CT (sometimes called μ-CT). Micro-CT scanners are similar to the clinical CT scanners used for human subjects, but scaled down for use on small animals, or small scale samples, with improved sensitivity. There are no real definitions in differences between micro and standard CT scanners, as well as the less commonly used intermediate mini-CT scanner [40].

Principle

CT-scanning works with the same fundamental principles as X-ray imaging, using X-ray electromagnetic rays to contrast tissues. CT scanners are an improvement on X-ray technology because they generate a 3D image of the tissue, by scanning cross sections across a sample. A computer then reconstructs the individual cross sectional images generated into usable images. The computer can also generate quantitative data CT scanning which reduce scatter problems [15, 41].

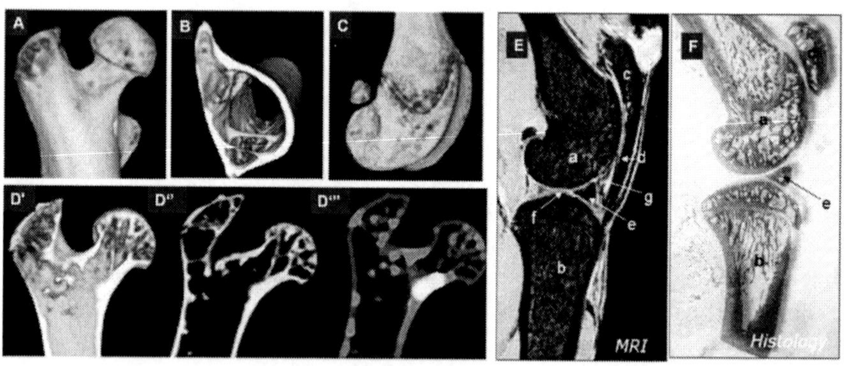

Figure 1. Micro-CT (A-D) and MRI (E & F) images of a rat (Wistar). A-C) Close views of the proximal epiphysis, metaphysis area and the femur condyles, respectively. D) Images displaying a sagittal 3D (D')and 2D cross section (D'') of the proximal epiphysis and a sagittal cross view showing a map of the bone thickness with higher density areas displayed as white (femoral neck)(D'''). E) 3D spin echo MR image of a rat knee *ex vivo* displaying the anatomical landmarks of the articular joint: a = femur condyle, b = tibia, c = patella, d = patellar ligament, e = meniscus, f = articular cartilage and g = intrapatellar fat pad. F) Histological image of the knee joint. (Tremoleda JL et al. EJNMMI Research 2011 1:11 doi:10.1186/2191-219X-1-11).

Micro-CT imaging began to be realised in the late 1980s, when the, still relatively new, CT technology was scaled down [42]. To scale the equipment down, a significant improvement in X-ray detector sensitivity was required. The advances in technology allowed the probing of dense structures, e.g. bone and implants, at a micrometer and even nanometer scale [41]. Preclinical micro-CT scanners harness an X-ray tube and a 2D X-ray detector to image a sample. Commercial micro-CT scanners work either by rotating the sample with a fixed source and detector, or by having a rotating source and detector image a fixed sample. For *in vivo* imaging, a fixed sample is typically preferred. For detailed analysis of individual bones many parameters such as beam strength, scanning time, animal fixation and how to keep the position of the area of tissue to be studied have to be optimised [43]. The technology is constantly being improved with changes to how data is collected and read for use in *in vivo* models [44].

Applications

Micro-CT has become the gold standard in imaging of small animal bones and micro-architecture (Figure 1A-D) [15]. Micro-CTs have been used for many applications in the non-invasive imaging of bone, which include, but are not limited to, research on skeleton formation [45], bone development and growth [46, 47], remodelling and regeneration [48, 49], cancer metastatic deposits [50] and fracture healing [51] as well as metabolic bone diseases [42]. Furthermore, rheumatoid arthritis modelling is a key area which has benefited from improvements in imaging quality; micro-CT has been highlighted as the best tool for the *in vivo* imaging of mouse arthritis models [42].

Today micro-CT images are routinely being used in research to non-invasively monitor and analyse implants, biomaterials and tissue formation. For example, R. Tanoue et al. (2013) used micro-CT images to monitor bone marrow stromal cells and fibroblasts forming bone in mouse models. They showed bone formation over an 8 week period with different cell types, and the data was confirmed with histological results afterwards [52].

Advantages and Disadvantages

Compared to other imaging technologies, such as the later explored MRI, micro-CT has powerful temporal and spatial resolution and is a considerably cheaper technology. It has been used extensively in research, as the wide range of applications listed shows, and is considered the gold standard for *in vivo* imaging for many areas of research.

One of the key problems associated with micro-CT is the long scanning times required for imaging. Despite being typically faster than MRI, the times can still be too long in practical terms. This is due to the problems with repeated anesthesia needed for long scanning times. Also, the breathing and small movements of the animal can affect imaging quality over long scan times. This can lead to difficulties in monitoring the dynamic processes of bone growth and regeneration, as the qualities of studies could be compromised [17]. Another concern with long scanning times, similar to those with 2D X-ray imaging, is the radiation associated with micro-CTs. Micro-CTs typically use more radiation than X-ray scanners, so attempts should be made to minimise radiation exposure, to keep studies unaffected [34, 35]. In principle, studies can take place over relatively long periods of time, assuming dosing problems are considered

Although contrast agents can improve the quality of imaging on soft tissues, it is still a major downside to using X-ray based imaging systems. Micro-CT cannot be used to full effect in some applications, such as early stages of bone healing processes [53].

Advances and Future Perspectives

CT technology scanning can be improved using a number of different methods [33] –

1) By combining X-ray CT images with other 2D images generated, such as radionucleotide-based images or even histological section images, to generate synergistic images. The process of this can be seen in later sections.
2) Contrast agents can be used to improve the contrast of radiographical imaging. For example, heavy elements can be attached to molecules of interest, or related molecules, to highlight areas of interest within the subject. Wong et al. (2013) used the heavy metal $GdCl_3$ for bone and used OsO_4 to stain the surrounding soft tissue structures, which resulted effectively imaged temporal bone in guinea pigs with micro-CT. This provided a contrast between two different tissues and helped create a detailed 3D rendered image [54].

3) By using additional parameters or methods to increase the sensitivity of the X-ray generated image, such as X-ray fluorescence imaging or analysis of scattered X-rays. Methods such as PET and SPECT can be combined with CT and will be discussed later [3, 42].

A newly developed R_mCT 3D micro X-ray CT scanner requires short, less potentially harmful, anesthetic times. This allowed the observation of new bone formation over 320 days. Prior studies had been unable to undertake such detailed long term studies because of the acquisition time problems [17].

Researchers always seek new way to improve existing technologies and discover alternative technologies where there are gaps in capabilities. To overcome the limitations of using X-ray and micro-CT, such as detailed soft tissue imaging, radiation concerns and anesthetic problems, other techniques such as Magnetic Resonance Imaging have been developed.

Magnetic Resonance Imaging (MRI)

Introduction and History

Another technique utilised for imaging bone *in vivo* is Magnetic Resonance Imaging (MRI) spectroscopy. MRI technology was developed in the early 1970s to meet a clinical need to image soft tissues. Alterations in Nuclear Magnetic Resonance (NMR) technology, which previously had only been used to characterise small molecules, lead to the development of MRI. In 2003 Paul Lauterbur and Peter Mansfield received the Nobel prize in physiology and medicine for the discovery of this breakthrough medical technology [55]. MRI is a non-invasive method which can be used to image organs such as bone for diagnosis, treatment and follow-up of treatments.

Principles

MRI is a NMR based technique, which exploits the magnetic properties of molecules by using a magnet field to excite them. Radio frequency pulses can then cause changes in those molecules, resulting in the induced spins then releasing their absorbed energy, as they return to their initial state. This release can then be detected, based on relaxation times, and used to construct MRI images [15, 47].

In theory, any atom with a net nucleus spin (an odd atomic weight or spin) can be imaged using MRI techniques. Biological samples are typically abundant in water, so by far the most established protocols for MRI are for ^{1}H atom imaging. Because of this MRI applications are usually in soft tissue imaging. With regards to bone, due to the phosphorous content of hydroxyapatite, the imaging of ^{31}P may also be a useful prospect [56]. Not particularly relevant for bone imaging, functional MRI (fMRI) is a special form of MRI which can image specific sections of the brain while performing tasks [53].

Applications

As a general rule MRI does not image bone well, because of its limited water content. ^{1}H imaging specifically does not paint a good picture of the actual structure of bone, particularly in the even lower water content trabecular bone (Figure 1E & F) [15]. This can be overcome by imaging the softer, higher water content tissues around bone, such as bone marrow. This creates a space in the exact shape of the bone, a negative image with the positive imaging of the soft tissues [47, 57]. However, such imaging only shows the shape of the bone, and does not provide any information on the actual composition or structure of the bone [58]. It is important to distinguish between those methods with generate data from the elemental analysis of bone itself, and those which look at the cavity from bone not being imaged by MRI [59].

Advantages and Disadvantages

MRI is a unique imaging technique because it can offer huge detail in soft tissue imaging, while still providing at least some information on bone. The ability to image detailed soft tissue changes, such as collection of synovial fluid, is particularly useful for arthritis models [65]. Another important advantage is the ability to tailor MRI imaging techniques to different materials, depending on their chemical composition. This could have uses in imaging implants or multiple tissues of interest [60].

Comparing to CT imaging, MRI has higher point-spread function leading to better imaging and a higher quality contrast between bone and marrow [59].

It also benefits from the fact that no ionising waves are used, which offers safety advantages over other methods such as X-ray and CT.

MRI technology is challenged when it comes to imaging small animals, despite the fact that the majority of the MRI studies on animals have been on mouse and rats, due to the practicalities of their use in research [56]. To achieve the high resolution necessary for MRI imaging of the very small bone structures of small animals there is normally a requirement of long acquisition times. To achieve the similar quality of imaging of bone, MRI requires much longer times than micro-CT scanning. Therefore, the necessary anesthetics have held back MRI as a bone imaging technique in live animal models [15]. In comparison, *in vivo* imaging of bone in human subjects, who don't require anesthetics, is actually more accurate. Thus, assumptions made from MRI images of human joints may mislead researchers in using MIR imaging in assessing animal joints [61].

Advances and Future Perspectives

One of the major challenges in generating high quality animal MRI images is the size of the radio coils which generate the radio frequency pulses. To overcome this, micro-MRI was developed for small subject image acquisition, restoration and processing. It is a scaled down version of a standard MRI scanner, so works with similar principles to micro-CT [57, 62].

Quantitative MRI options have also been developed greatly over the last 15 years and can lead to accurate data on bone mass, structure and function, through a number of different methods [59]. Over the last few years, high field quantitative MRI has been developed to allow imaging the bones and joints in small animal. This has been used to monitor disease models in rats [63] and guinea pigs [64]. A number of studies showed that MRI is comparable to mico-CT, and the 'gold standard' of histology, for even very early changes in rat *in vivo* models of inflammatory arthritis.

To date, MRI is routinely used models to investigate the effect of degenerative diseases such as osteoarthritis and rheumatoid arthritis; however, often with a focus on cartilage, although bone is also usually imaged in the process [28, 29]. Although high field quantitative MRI originally only generated data on the easier to image peripheral skeleton, technology refinements mean that the rest of the skeleton can be imaged to a good resolution [66]. Moreover, MRI and micro-CT have been used for *in vivo* drug testing of rat models of posttraumatic secondary osteoarthritis [67].

Different pulse sequences can be used to obtain more realistic time frames, giving sufficient resolution to image small animal bones. These include 3D gradient-echo sequences, which allow for a shorter acquisition times. Detailed joint analysis of rats has been achieved in this way, with comparable results to histological analysis [61]. Alterations in the pulse sequences and echo times can be implemented and specifically tailored to detect signals from tissues such as bone. Ultra-short echo-time (UTE) radial acquisition MRI can offer alternative imaging capabilities, allowing imaging of different types of bone and tissues such as the periosteum [60, 68].

Another technique employed to improve the MRI imaging of bone is that of water- and fat- suppressed proton projection imaging (WASPI). WASPI utilises solid state MRI, which uses a high intensity short duration pulse to fully excite a signal from tissues, i.e. bone. This can then have the signals from fluid suppression subtracted, which generates images of pure bone. These can also be used to calculate bone density and has been shown to be effective in human and pig models [58].

Contrast agents are also used to improve MRI. Most research is utilises the Gd(III) ion, because of its long spin relaxation time and high magnetic moment [69]. When encapsulated in complexes, Gd(III) along with other Lanthanide (III) ions, can become safe to use as an MRI contrasting agent. A whole plethora of contrast agents are available which can accelerate the relaxation times of water protons which can enhance the contrast and improve MRI images of bone [70].

PET and SPECT Nuclear Imaging Technologies

Introduction and History

In a similar vein to MRI, emission tomography technologies are nuclear imaging techniques which can depict biological tissue. These include positron emission tomography (PET) and single-photon emission computed tomography (SPECT).

The concept of emission and transmission tomography was first introduced by David E. Kuhl et al. in the 1950s, when the radioisotope technetium-99m (^{99m}Tc) was used to highlight areas of the brain in scanning. Based on this technology, SPECT was developed in the 1960s and PET technology was fully developed in the late 1970s. Radiotracer molecules are often attached to other compounds, such as sodium fluoride. The first application of sodium fluoride labelled with ^{18}F for imaging of bone was back in 1962. In the 1970s this was mostly replaced by the ^{99}Tc labelled diphosphate compounds. However, these ^{99}Tc imaging agents are relatively wide targeting and have low levels of specificity. PET imaging was known to have advantages over SPECT; however, there were associated research reimbursement issues with PET and as a result it was only used as a research tool in the early 1990s. Today both are now used extensively both as a research tool and in clinical settings [71–73].

Principles

PET and SPECT are based on the detection of specific molecules; in the case of SPECT gamma photons released by decaying radioisotopes; for PET the emission of positrons from decaying radioisotopes. These radiotracer molecules are specially designed to concentrate in a specific area of interest in the subject, leading to a high concentration of emission, which is then read by a lead or tungsten collimator [53].

The technology is designed to utilise imaging agents, made of radioisotopes attached to other molecules to image areas of interest based on the signals the isotopes emit. While PET results are impressive, ^{99}Tc SPECT is still a relevant technology for imaging of bone [72, 73]. ^{68}Ga PET is a commonly used alternative to ^{18}F PET, as there is much potential in the combination of bisphosphonates and ligands such as the macrocyclic DOTA [73, 74].

When bone is being damaged or deposited in tumour formation, hydroxyapatite crystals can become exposed, and can be targeted by ^{99}Tc labelled methylene diphosphate or hydroxyl methylene diphosphate. Then the bone can be imaged to visualise any abnormalities such as a stress fractures [16].

Practically, the imaging agents are injected into the blood of subjects and any tracer unbound in the blood can then be taken up by bone. How such agents are taken up by the bone depends on the agent, the diffusion through capillaries, and how the bone is forming and remodelling. It is understood that bisphosphonates, which used with labels such as ^{68}Ga and ^{99}Tc are one of the most researched compounds in this field, bind to hydroxyapatite which is deposited and exposed in bone remodelling [73, 75]. ^{18}F labelled fluoride is absorbed onto the bone surface from the blood. Other agents such as ^{68}GaBPAMD are thought to be taken up by osteoclasts, and thus are more suited to imaging areas with high levels of osteoclasts, such as cancerous lesions. Therefore, it is important to consider the method of uptake of the agent when choosing imaging agents [76].

Applications

These techniques facilitate academic and industrial research for drug discovery and evaluation purposes, and have neurological, cardiovascular and oncological research applications [6]. More importantly, emission tomography technologies have been extensively used in bone imaging for investigating bone metatheses and tumours, allowing whole skeletons to be imaged. Also, importantly, the detection can be performed quantitatively (Figure 2B) [15]. For the *in vivo* imaging of bone, studies have been undertaken imaging fractures [16], analysing detailed microdamage [78], and monitoring bone turnover [77] have been undertaken.

In an *in vivo* study with mice, whole mouse skeletons were imaged to by identifying ^{125}I labelled bone-targeted copolymers. This was found to particularly highlight sites of high bone turnover [77].

Advantages and Disadvantages

These imaging technologies do not achieve the resolution of other techniques such as MRI or micro-CT, but they can provide detailed information on physiological and metabolic processes in real time, and are often used in conjunction with other imaging technologies. They have the potential to be low cost, of broad availability and can be tailored and optimised for different applications based on the half-life and designed specificity of agents [6].

An advantage of these technologies is, while resolution can be questionable, ^{18}F labelled NaF PET and ^{99m}Tc SPECT can be used to generate accurate quantitative data [72]. For example, PET and ^{18}F labelled NaF have been used as a tracer to detect bone microdamage in rat models, including details about the type and cause of the damage. The results can detect very sensitive and hard to quantify changes in bone architecture [78].

PET is reported to be superior to SPECT for imaging bone tissue [74]. PET is well suited for animal imaging as it has a significantly higher sensitivity and there are greater possibilities for incorporation of positron labels into biomolecules. SPECT is a relatively low sensitivity imaging technique, which often cannot generate high quality structural images of bone.. The collimator used for SPECT imaging makes it a relatively low sensitivity imaging technique. However, in comparison to PET it has been well researched and the radiotracer compounds are relatively easy to obtain. While PET imaging may be more sensitive, SPECT has a better spatial resolution than PET and it can be used to image multiple probes utilising different isotope labels, allowing simultaneous study of different events or structures [6, 71]. Moreover, SPECT can be used to generate reasonably detailed pictures of bone for studying biological processes at a molecular and cellular level, which is unparalleled [53].

Currently these technologies are primarily limited by low resolutions and minimal research having been undertaken into their uses. These imaging agents can be somewhat limited in their specificity, availability and production. The safety, stability and toxicology of any imaging agents used must always be considered when designing agents.

Advances and Future Perspectives

Recently, a novel macrocyclic system was developed, which utilises a polymer and the ^{68}Ga radioisotope for bone imaging. This imaging agent can bind to bone to improve the stability and potential applications of PET [79].

Nanomedicine technology can be exploited to target areas of diseased bone for a synergistic process of imaging and treating bone disease. To this end, bisphosphonates have been used in many of the medical imaging technologies, and have been proven in clinical trials to have a therapeutic use in increasing bone strength [75]. Also, polymers can be specifically designed to target bone and release agents for bone imaging, and/or therapeutics. These ideas are relatively new and the applications are currently limited [80].

These compounds may have uses in cancer therapies, as there is also potential to synergistically treat and image bone metatheses when therapeutic nucleotides, such as ^{177}Lu are combined with already established technologies such as the ^{68}Ga-PET agents. There is the potential to combine these with more established agents such as DOTA-bisphosphonates, with significant commercial and practical benefits [74]. A relatively unexplored isotope for bone PET imaging is ^{64}Cu, which has been proven to be useful in a small animal model as a potentially useful combined therapy and emitter. Combined with bifunctional chelator molecules, they could be used for bone cancer treatments and imaging [32].

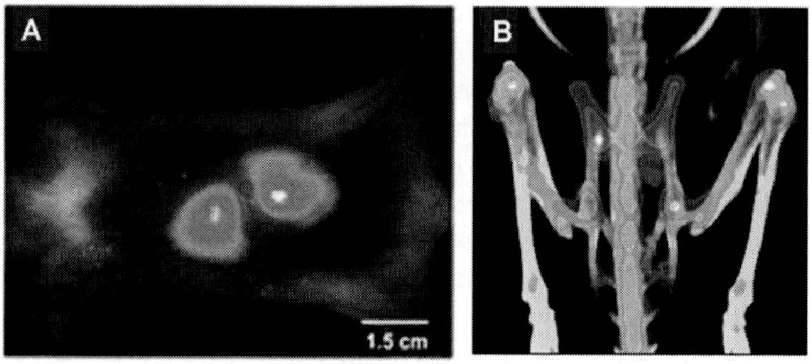

Figure 2. Fluorescent optical imaging for *in vivo* monitoring (A) and the combination of micro-SPECT with micro-CT images of bone (B). A) Multispectral images of the TRITC labelled scaffolds after implantation in MF1 mice (Cunha-Reis C et al. JTERM 2013 doi: 10.1002/term.494). B) Micro-SPECT/CT images of the posterior quarter of the mouse, showing the uptake in the hip joint (femur and sacrum) and the knee joints . (Tremoleda JL et al. EJNMMI Research 2011 1:11 doi:10.1186/2191-219X-1-11).

Optical Imaging Technologies – Fluorescence and Bioluminescence

Introduction and History

There is currently an ongoing revolution in the field of *in vivo* optical imaging. *Optical* imaging technologies found their roots in bench top bioluminescence kits, using selected substrates to monitor changes in cells. Such technologies found themselves at the forefront of research at the turn of the century [81], and moved into *in vivo* applications shortly after [82]. These tools are rapidly being developed to be powerful, detailed, real time, non-invasive *in vivo* imaging tools. The field is still relatively new, especially when compared to the well-established techniques discussed before.

Fluorescence

Principles

The principle behind fluorescence technology is similar to that of PET and SPECT. These technologies monitor light emission from fluorophores which are bound to a substrate (Figure 2A). These substrates are designed to target an area of interest, such as a specific cell type [8]. Fluorescence imaging works by using an external excitation wave at a set wavelength to excite the fluorophores. This causes the fluorophore to emit photons which, because they are at a different wavelength to the excitation wave, can be imaged [83].

Non-specific fluorophores can be designed to image areas where a process such as inflammation is taking place. Also, they can be part of specific targeting systems, such as when tagged to antibodies which bind to specific cells, molecules and metabolic pathways or tagged to specific reporter proteins to image gene expression [15].

Applications

This technology has been used to study bone formation and resorption *in vivo* since 2001. A fluorophore bound to bisphosphonate will bind to the exposed hydroxyapatite in the regions of high bone turnover and resulting fluorescence can be measured once excited [84]. The benefits of, and concerns with, bisphosphonate probes have been explored in the SPECT/PET section [75]. Recently, more probes have been developed to monitor how these are deposited in *in vivo* models [85], such as the commercially available OsteoSense® (Caliper® Life Science). This is a probe which comprises of a bisphosphonate ligand and a far-red fluorescent pamidronate, which has been shown to be potentially useful in the non-invasive monitoring of bone cancers, bone fractures and healing in mouse models [86]. Other commercial probes include BoneTag™ (LI-COR® Biosciences) and the fluorescently labelled alendronate (Caliper® Life Sciences). Alendronate is a bisphosphonate similar to OsteoSense®, but BoneTag™ is a fluorescently labelled tetracyclic device. They are available in a number of different excitation and emission wavelengths, allowing tailoring of systems [83].

Furthermore, rheumatoid arthritis often produces specific cytokines and proteins for which fluorescent probes or antibodies can be designed to bind to the area of interest, resulting in fluorescent imaging of the arthritic mouse joint. While this is not imaging bone directly it can provide information about arthritis, and is quantitative. It is thought these methods may be superior in some respects to the more conventional techniques of MRI and X-ray diagnosis, because it gives a much earlier indicator of the disease [87, 88].

Advantages and Disadvantages

These technologies developed due to a need to improve on agents such as those used for SPECT. The penetration of photons generated from fluorophores through tissues is higher than that of gamma rays. This is coupled with the fact that photos scatter less when travelling through tissues. Also, there is little background noise as tissue's autofluorescence and absorption of fluorescence is low, especially if near-red fluorescence light is used over green [83, 84]. Other advantages of using fluorescent probes over the radioactive bone tracers discussed earlier include the fact there is less concern about probes decaying over storage time, and radioactive capable infrastructure is not necessary. More importantly, fluorescent imaging technologies require shorter scan times, a major advantage when employing non-invasive in *in vivo* models [83].

Fluorescence imaging has similar disadvantages to PET and SPECT, as they have low a resolution, especially when compared to other technologies such as micro-CT [74].

Advances and Future Perspectives

The technology has recently advanced to be able to generate 3D images of fluorescent probes, using Fluorescent Molecular Tomography (FMT). FMT generates images from small illuminations across multiple points in the sample, across a pre-set grid. This generates data from multiple positions, and along with measurements of light propagation through the tissue, can be used to construct a 3D distribution pattern. In the 2D technology a wide illumination simply illuminates the sample and the resulting excitation is measured [8, 89].

F. Lambers et al. (2013) combined this technology with micro-CT to monitor *in vivo* bone responses to loading in mice models [8]. Studies such as these are likely to be the future of these technologies, as combination with other imaging to gives a much better overall picture.

Recent research has measured osteoclast activity using different methods. For example, Cathepsin K-induced fluorescence probe using a Cy5.5 fluorophore were used to image early signs of bone loss *in vivo.* This technology has potential advantages over the aforementioned bisphosphonate technologies, which may have difficulty differentiating between area of high hydroxyapatite density and exposed hydroxyapatite in osteolytic areas [74]. Cathepsin K activity is believed to be a good marker of very early bone loss, so it could potentially be combined with fluorescent probes to be very powerful tool to image bone *in vivo* [90].

Bioluminescence

Principles

Bioluminescent technology is based on the principles of enzymatic reactions releasing photons. It is a naturally occurring phenomenon seen in fireflies and other organisms.

Basically, molecules can be transfected into cells of interest, such as cancer cells, and then used to monitor the cell's progress *in vivo*. To date, luciferase proteins from fireflies [91] and 'Green Fluorescent Protein' (GFP) [92] are the most commonly used in imaging.

Applications

In research, bioluminescent is most commonly utilised in gene reporter assays in tests for the presence of a substrate. But this technology can also be utilised for in non-invasive *in vivo* imaging. The technology is very limited at the moment, with very few examples of applications, especially in bone tissue imaging [15].

Metastatic deposits in mice bone marrow are notoriously hard to monitor using conventional methods. Bioluminescence allows the sensitive imaging of tumour growth in bone marrow from an early stage [93].

In the field of cell-based therapy and tissue engineering, bioluminescence imaging can be used to monitor cell's underlying events such as cell migration, proliferation and differentiation *in vivo*. This is especially useful as knowledge is limited on the events that follow implantation of cells. With careful system design a number of different promoters can be utilised, depending on the desired outcome. Both the firefly luciferase and GFP systems can be used to track stem cells in bone healing models [94]. Systems can be designed where a promoter transgene such as 2.3Col1a1 can drive bioluminescent biomarkers to visualise bone tissues [95]. Bioluminescent imaging can be used to track how mesenchymal stem cells migrate to fracture sites *in vivo* and how growth factors and changes to stem cell populations can affect such processes [96]. More recently osteogenic differentiation of human bone marrow cells in a mouse defect model [94].

Advantages and Disadvantages

This technology has the advantage of being highly specific for the genes of interest, typically having a low background signal, and genes can be studied non-invasively over the whole lifetime of an animal [15].

However, this technology has not been well researched and the resolution of the images are relatively low. Thus, it is probably a technology which will best find itself combined with other techniques such as mirco-CT.

Advances and Future Perspectives

Bioluminescence is a relatively newly realised technology but has quickly advanced into quantitative studies. This technology can be used to quantitatively and reliably monitor skeleton growth and repair in real time. This also has the potential to be used for investigating the effects of drugs or other treatments on the skeleton [97]. Furthermore, bioluminescence can be a useful tool to investigate any proteins which may be relevant to skeletal development or repair. For example, an osteocalcin luciferase system was used to monitor skeletal development and repair in transgenic mice. This has the potential to be utilised in investigating the effects of drugs, foods, age or other treatments on the skeleton [9, 97]. Osteolysis is a major problem in joint implants and this can be imaged using bioluminescence, by detecting the luminescence generated from activation of inflammatory response factors, [98] or by monitoring macrophage migration to the sites of wear particles [99].

Ultrasound

Introduction and History

Ultrasound, also known as Ultrasonography or Sonography, was first produced by a whistle experiment conducted by Sir Francis Galton in 1893. The first applications of ultrasound in bone imaging were in the 1950s, where tibia bone fractures were explored. Since then ultrasound has been routinely used for assessment of bone *in vivo*, both in human and animal models. The technology was massively improved with the development of Quantitative Ultrasound (QUS) in the 1980s, first used for monitoring osteoporosis [100]. Because of its integral role in osteoporosis research, the discovery has been highlighted by UK Universities as one of the top "100 discoveries and developments in UK Universities that have changed the world" [101].

Principles

An ultrasound wave is an oscillating sound pressure wave with a frequency greater than the upper limit of the human hearing range. Ultrasound generates information about tissues based on the amount of ultrasound waves that are transmitted and reflected by the tissue [53].

Applications

Ultrasound has been used for medical imaging for more than 50 years. The majority of literature published on ultrasound uses in bone imaging are for bone density analysis. It is often employed in solid organ and soft tissue imaging scenarios, to investigate diseases and organ pathology. Also, ultrasound can be especially useful for use in rheumatoid arthritis models, such as in drug trials [13, 53].

A number of studies have shown that ultrasound can be used for *in vivo* imaging to monitor bone fracture healing processes [14, 102], the changes of the joint's structure during the development of osteoarthritis [26, 27], bone mineral density [103], and cartilage and subchondral bone *in vivo* [104]. Recently, ultrasound has been established as the most reliable method for assessing mechanical quality of bones for use in dental work in *in vivo* models [105–107].

The reason for ultrasound mainly being used in bone density studies is the high levels of wave loss resulting from transitions between soft and hard tissues. This results in poor *in vivo* imaging of the skeleton. This issue is being worked on with new technologies such as densitometers, which can utilise both fast and slow longitudinal waves to image bone, with results comparable to micro-CT in human subjects [108].

For fracture healing, there are a number of non-invasive methods which can provide quantitative data of healing, such as bone densitometry, vibrational analysis, acoustic emission and the use of attached strain gauges. However, these are all reasonably archaic technologies with practical drawbacks. Therefore, ultrasound technology has the potential to be superior for imaging of fracture healing models [14].

Advantages and Disadvantages

Ultrasound is a very useful tool for *in vivo* imaging because it is non-invasive, relatively low cost, and provides detailed information on *in vivo* subjects in real-time. Also ultrasound devices are usually portable. In medical scenarios, properly performed ultrasound poses no known risks to the patient. Ultrasound is very effective for generating information such as density and fracture healing, providing data in different forms to the other techniques discussed [109].

As mentioned above, ultrasound imaging is mainly used for density studies and it is currently poor for actually generating images of bone compared to other techniques such as micro-CT [108].

Advances and Future Perspectives

In general, the ultrasound wave frequencies are typically between 3 and 50 MHz. But the ultrasound image can be further enhanced by using ultrahigh frequencies between 20MHz and 100 MHz, which allow sufficient resolution to image very fine detailed structures, such as the reproductive system [110]. This technique is sometimes called Ultrasound Biomicroscopy, and is an advance on the standard ultrasound technology, attempting to improve on the relatively poor imaging resolution of ultrasound.

Conclusion

This chapter has covered brief histories, principles, applications, advantages, disadvantages and recent developments of the tools available for the *in vivo* imaging of bone. Covered were X-ray, micro computed tomography, magnetic resonance imaging, SPECT/PET nuclear imaging, fluorescence, bioluminescent and ultrasound technologies.

The use of animal models is essential on so many levels of research. Being able to image these non-invasively is fundamental in generating biologically significant results. The *in vivo* modelling of bone has undergone much research and can be undertaken effectively utilising a number of different methods. As technologies become more affordable and widely available, the combination of different techniques is becoming more and more common place in publications [6, 8, 13]. They ability to overlay images from different technologies on one another is very powerful. However, it is important to choose the proper methods for the model. Improvements to the currently available imaging systems and development of new methods will enhance the quality of the studies with economic, research quality and ethical implications.

References

[1] Rodan GA, Martin JT. Therapeutic Approaches to Bone Diseases. *Science*. 2000 Sep 1;289(5484):1508–14.

[2] Spiegel P. The first clinical X-ray made in America--100 years. *American journal of roentgenology*. 1995;164(1):241–3.

[3] Chen H, Rogalski MM, Anker JN. Advances in functional X-ray imaging techniques and contrast agents. *Physical chemistry chemical physics*. 2012 Oct 21;14(39):13469–86.

[4] Winkelmann CT, Figueroa SD, Sieckman GL, Rold TL, Hoffman TJ. Non-invasive microCT imaging characterization and in vivo targeting of BB2 receptor expression of a PC-3 bone metastasis model. *Molecular imaging and biology*. 2012 Dec;14(6):667–75.

[5] Long C, Bulte J. In vivo tracking of cellular therapeutics using magnetic resonance imaging. *Expert Opinion on Biological Therapy*. 2009; 9(3):293–306.

[6] Franc BL, Acton PD, Mari C, Hasegawa BH. Small-animal SPECT and SPECT/CT: important tools for preclinical investigation. *Journal of nuclear medicine*. 2008 Oct;49(10):1651–63.

[7] Kaufman JJ, Einhorn TA. Perspectives Ultrasound Assessment of Bone. *Journal of bone and mineral research*. 1993;8(5):517–25.

[8] Lambers FM, Stuker F, Weigt C, Kuhn G, Koch K, Schulte FA, et al. Longitudinal in vivo imaging of bone formation and resorption using fluorescence molecular tomography. *Bone*. Elsevier Inc.; 2013 Feb; 52(2):587–95.

[9] Nakanishi T, Kokubun K, Oda H, Aoki M, Soma A, Taniguchi M, et al. Bioluminescence imaging of bone formation using hairless osteocalcin-luciferase transgenic mice. *Bone*. Elsevier Inc.; 2012 Sep;51(3):369–75.

[10] Xiadou W, Nyman JS, Reyes M, Dong X, Leng H, Athanasiou KA. Fundamental Biomechanics in Bone Tissue Engineering. Morgan and Claypool Publishers; 2010. p. 230.

[11] Jones E, Yang X. Mesenchymal stem cells and bone regeneration: current status. *Injury*.; 2011 Jun;42(6):562–8.

[12] Horner E, Kirkham J, Yang XB. Basic Science/Animal Models. In: Polak J et al., editor. Advances in Tissue Engineering. 1st ed. London: Imperial College Press; 2008. p. 763–79.

[13] Beckmann N, Kneuer R. In vivo mouse imaging and spectroscopy in drug discovery. *NMR in Biomedicine*. 2007;20:154–85.

[14] Protopappas VC, Vavva MG, Fotiadis DI, Malizos KN. Ultrasonic monitoring of bone fracture healing. *IEEE transactions on ultrasonics, ferroelectrics, and frequency control*. 2008 Jan;55(6):1243–55.

[15] Tremoleda JL, Khalil M, Gompels LL, Wylezinska-Arridge M, Vincent T, Gsell W. Imaging technologies for preclinical models of bone and joint disorders. *EJNMMI research*. 2011 Jan;1(1):11.

[16] Arkader A, Morris CD. Lymphatic spread of pagetic osteogenic sarcoma detected by bone scan. *Cancer imaging*. 2008 Jan;8:131–4.

[17] Sato Y, Observation L, Bone E, Hayashi T, Hamazima S, Asakura M. Original Long-Term Observation of Ectopic Bone Formation Using In Vivo Microcomputed Tomography. *Journal of Hard Tissue Biology*. 2013;22(3):343–550.

[18] Hessenbruch A. A brief history of x-rays. *Endeavour*. 2002 Dec; 26(4):137–41.

[19] Junqueira LC, Carneiro J. Junqueira's Basic Histology: Text and Atlas. 11th ed. New York: McGraw-Hill Medical; 2005.

[20] Bull S. Skeletal Radiography: A Concise Introduction to Projection Radiography. 2nd Rev ed. Toolkit Publications; 2005. p. 1–205.

[21] Bilezikian JP, Raisz LG, Martin TJ. Principles of Bone Biology. 3rd ed. San Diego: Academic Press inc Elsevier Science; 2008.

[22] Bueno EM, Glowacki J. Biological Foundations for Skeletal Tissue Engineering. *Synthesis Lectures on Tissue Engineering*.; 2011;3(1):p. 1–220.

[23] Marieb EN. Human Anatomy and Physiology. 4th ed. San Francisco City: Benjamin-Cummings Publishing Company; 1997.

[24] Bartel DL, Davy DT, Keaveny TM. Orthopaedic Biomechanics: Mechanics and Design in Musculoskeletal Systems. *Pearson Education;* 2006. p. 1–384.

[25] Yang Y-Q, Tan Y-Y, Wong R, Wenden A, Zhang L-K, Rabie a BM. The role of vascular endothelial growth factor in ossification. *International journal of oral science*. 2012 Jun;4(2):64–8.

[26] Podlipská J, Koski JM, Pulkkinen P, Saarakkala S. In vivo quantitative ultrasound image analysis of femoral subchondral bone in knee osteoarthritis. *The Scientific World Journal*. 2013 Jan;2013:182562.

[27] Iagnocco A. Imaging the joint in osteoarthritis: a place for ultrasound? Best practice & research. *Clinical rheumatology*. 2010 Feb;24(1):27–38.

[28] Laurent D, O'Byrne E, Wasvary J, Pellas TC. In vivo MRI of cartilage pathogenesis in surgical models of osteoarthritis. *Skeletal radiology*. 2006 Aug;35(8):555–64.

[29] Dao TT, Pouletaut P, Goebel J-C, Pinzano a., Gillet P, Ho Ba Tho MC. In vivo characterization of morphological properties and contact areas of the rat cartilage derived from high-resolution MRI. *Irbm*. 2011 Jun;32(3):204–13.

[30] Seibert JA. X-ray imaging physics for nuclear medicine technologists. Part 1: Basic principles of x-ray production. *Journal of nuclear medicine technology*. 2004 Sep;32(3):139–47.

[31] Attwood D. Soft X-Rays and Extreme Ultraviolet Radiation. 1st ed. Cambridge: Cambridge University Press; 2007. p. 1–504.

[32] Sprague JE, Kitaura H, Zou W, Ye Y, Achilefu S, Weilbaecher KN, et al. Noninvasive imaging of osteoclasts in parathyroid hormone-induced osteolysis using a 64Cu-labeled RGD peptide. *Journal of nuclear medicine*. 2007 Feb;48(2):311–8.

[33] Ritman EL. Molecular imaging in small animals--roles for micro-CT. Journal of cellular biochemistry. *Supplement*. 2002;39(October):116–24.

[34] Kadhim M, Salomaa S, Wright E, Hildebrandt G, Belyakov O V, Prise KM, et al. Non-targeted effects of ionising radiation-Implications for low dose risk. *Mutation research.* 2013;752(2):84–98.
[35] Boone JM, Velazquez O, Cherry SR. Small-animal X-ray dose from micro-CT. *Molecular imaging*. 2004 Jul;3(3):149–58.
[36] Nagy TR, Clair a L. Precision and accuracy of dual-energy X-ray absorptiometry for determining in vivo body composition of mice. *Obesity research.* 2000 Aug;8(5):392–8.
[37] Swennen Q, Janssens GPJ, Geers R, Decuypere E, Buyse J. Validation of dual-energy x-ray absorptiometry for determining in vivo body composition of chickens. *Poultry science*. 2004 Aug;83(8):1348–57.
[38] Bolotin HH. Inaccuracies inherent in dual-energy X-ray absorptiometry in vivo bone mineral densitometry may flaw osteopenic/osteoporotic interpretations and mislead assessment of antiresorptive therapy effectiveness. *Bone*. 2001 May;28(5):548–55.
[39] Hainfeld JF, Slatkin DN, Focella TM, Smilowitz HM. Gold nanoparticles: a new X-ray contrast agent. *The British journal of radiology*. 2006 Mar;79(939):248–53.
[40] Bartling S, Stiller W, Semmler W, Kiessling F. Small Animal Computed Tomography Imaging. *Current Medical Imaging Reviews*. 2007 Feb 1;3(1):45–59.
[41] Goldman LW. Principles of CT and CT technology. *Journal of nuclear medicine technology*. 2007 Sep;35(3):115–28; quiz 129–30.
[42] Schambach SJ, Bag S, Schilling L, Groden C, Brockmann M a. Application of micro-CT in small animal imaging. *Methods*. 2010 Jan;50(1):2–13.
[43] Arentsen L, Hui S. Characterization of rotating gantry micro-CT configuration for the in vivo evaluation of murine trabecular bone. *Microscopy and microanalysis*. 2013 Aug; 19(4):907–13.
[44] Johnston SM, Johnson GA, Badea CT. Geometric calibration for a dual tube/detector micro-CT system. *Medical Physics*. 2008;35(5):1820.
[45] Guldberg RE, Lin ASP, Coleman R, Robertson G, Duvall C. Microcomputed tomography imaging of skeletal development and growth. Birth defects research. Part C, *Embryo today*: reviews. 2004 Sep;72(3):250–9.
[46] David V, Laroche N, Boudignon B, Lafage-Proust M-H, Alexandre C, Ruegsegger P, et al. Noninvasive in vivo monitoring of bone architecture alterations in hindlimb-unloaded female rats using novel

three-dimensional microcomputed tomography. *Journal of bone and mineral research*. 2003 Sep;18(9):1622–31.

[47] Jiang Y, Zhao J, White DL, Genant HK. Micro CT and Micro MR imaging of 3D architecture of animal skeleton. Journal of musculoskeletal & neuronal interactions. 2000 Sep;1(1):45–51.

[48] Waarsing JH, Day JS, Weinans H. Longitudinal micro-CT scans to evaluate bone architecture. *Journal of musculoskeletal & neuronal interactions*. 2005;5(4):310–2.

[49] Freeman T a, Patel P, Parvizi J, Antoci V, Shapiro IM. Micro-CT analysis with multiple thresholds allows detection of bone formation and resorption during ultrasound-treated fracture healing. *Journal of orthopaedic research*. 2009 May;27(5):673–9.

[50] Patel V, Issever AS, Burghardt A, Laib A, Ries M, Majumdar S. MicroCT evaluation of normal and osteoarthritic bone structure in human knee specimens. *Journal of orthopaedic research*. 2003 Jan;21(1):6–13.

[51] Nyman JS, Munoz S, Jadhav S, Mansour A, Yoshii T, Mundy GR, et al. Quantitative measures of femoral fracture repair in rats derived by micro-computed tomography. *Journal of biomechanics*. 2009 May 11;42(7):891–7.

[52] Tanoue R, Ohta K, Ogasawara S, Yano H, Kusukawa J, Nakamura K. Bone marrow stromal cells can cause subcutaneous fibroblasts to differentiate into osteocytes in a physically stable spatial microenvironment in rats. *Acta histochemica*. 2013 Jun;115(5):512–8.

[53] Kagadis GC, Loudos G, Katsanos K, Langer SG, Nikiforidis GC. In vivo small animal imaging: Current status and future prospects. *Medical Physics*. 2010;37(12):6421–42.

[54] Wong CC, Curthoys IS, O'Leary SJ, Jones AS. Heavy metal staining, a comparative assessment of gadolinium chloride and osmium tetroxide for inner ear labyrinthine contrast enhancement using X-ray microtomography. *Acta oto-laryngologica*. 2013 Jan;133(1):22–7.

[55] Pearson H. Magnetic pioneers net Nobel for putting medicine in the picture. *Nature*. 2003;425(October):2003.

[56] Heerschap A, Sommers MG, in 't Zandt HJA, Renema WKJ, Veltien AA, Klomp DWJ. Nuclear magnetic resonance in laboratory animals. *Methods in enzymology*. 2004 Jan;385(2001):41–63.

[57] Takahashi M, Wehrli FW, Hilaire L, Zemel BS, Hwang SN. In vivo NMR microscopy allows short-term serial assessment of multiple skeletal implications of corticosteroid exposure. *Proceedings of the*

National Academy of Sciences of the United States of America. 2002 Apr 2;99(7):4574–9.

[58] Wu Y, Hrovat MI, Ackerman JL, Reese TG, Cao H, Ecklund K, et al. Bone matrix imaged in vivo by water- and fat-suppressed proton projection MRI (WASPI) of animal and human subjects. *Journal of magnetic resonance imaging*. 2010 Apr;31(4):954–63.

[59] Wehrli FW, Song HK, Saha PK, Wright AC. Quantitative MRI for the assessment of bone structure and function. *NMR in Biomedicine*. 2006;19:731–64.

[60] Anumula S, Wehrli SL, Magland J, Wright a C, Wehrli FW. Ultra-short echo-time MRI detects changes in bone mineralization and water content in OVX rat bone in response to alendronate treatment. *Bone*. 2010 May;46(5):1391–9.

[61] Wang H-H, Wang Y-XJ, Griffith JF, Sun Y-L, Zhang G, Chan C-W, et al. Pitfalls in interpreting rat knee joint magnetic resonance images and their histological correlation. *Acta radiologica*. 2009 Nov;50(9):1042–8.

[62] Hwang S, Wehrli F. Estimating voxel volume fractions of trabecular bone on the basis of magnetic resonance images acquired in vivo. *International journal of imaging systems and technology*. 1999;10(2):186–98.

[63] Faure P, Doan B-T, Beloeil J-C. In-vivo high resolution three-dimensional MRI studies of rat joints at 7 T. *NMR in biomedicine*. 2003 Dec; 16(8):484–93.

[64] Watson P, Carpenter T, Hall L, Tyler J. MR protocols for imaging the guinea pig knee. *Magnetic resonance imaging*. 1997;15(8):957–70.

[65] Lee S-W, Greve JM, Leaffer D, Lollini L, Bailey P, Gold GE, et al. Early findings of small-animal MRI and small-animal computed tomography correlate with histological changes in a rat model of rheumatoid arthritis. *NMR in Biomedicine*. 2008;21:527–36.

[66] Patsch JM, Burghardt AJ, Kazakia G, Majumdar S. Noninvasive imaging of bone microarchitecture. *Annals of the New York Academy of Sciences*. 2011 Dec;1240:77–87.

[67] Jones MD, Tran CW, Li G, Maksymowych WP, Zernicke RF, Doschak MR. In vivo microfocal computed tomography and micro-magnetic resonance imaging evaluation of antiresorptive and antiinflammatory drugs as preventive treatments of osteoarthritis in the rat. *Arthritis and rheumatism*. 2010 Sep;62(9):2726–35.

[68] Tyler DJ, Robson MD, Henkelman RM, Young IR, Bydder GM. Magnetic resonance imaging with ultrashort TE (UTE) PULSE

sequences: technical considerations. *Journal of magnetic resonance imaging*. 2007 Feb; 25(2):279–89.

[69] Caravan P, Ellison JJ, McMurry TJ, Lauffer RB. Gadolinium(III) Chelates as MRI Contrast Agents: Structure, Dynamics, and Applications. *Chemical reviews*. 1999 Sep 8;99(9):2293–352.

[70] James Ratnakar S, Arockia Samy N, Alexander V. A new potential contrast agent for magnetic resonance imaging: Synthesis and relaxivity studies of a gadolinium(III) complex of glucose-6-phosphate conjugated 1, 4, 7, 10-tetraazacyclododecane-1, 4, 7-triacetic acid. *Polyhedron*. 2012 May;38(1):1–6.

[71] Blake P, Johnson B, VanMeter J. Positron emission tomography (PET) and single photon emission computed tomography (SPECT): clinical applications. *Journal of Neuro-Ophthalmology*. 2003;23(1):34–41.

[72] Blake GM, Park-Holohan SJ, Cook GJ, Fogelman I. Quantitative studies of bone with the use of 18F-fluoride and 99mTc-methylene diphosphonate. *Seminars in nuclear medicine*. 2001 Jan;31(1):28–49.

[73] Wong KK, Piert M. Dynamic bone imaging with 99mTc-labeled diphosphonates and 18F-NaF: mechanisms and applications. *Journal of nuclear medicine*. 2013 Apr;54(4):590–9.

[74] Meckel M, Fellner M, Thieme N, Bergmann R, Kubicek V, Rösch F. In vivo comparison of DOTA based (68)Ga-labelled bisphosphonates for bone imaging in non-tumour models. *Nuclear medicine and biology*. 2013 Aug;40(6):823–30.

[75] Papapoulos SE. Bisphosphonates: how do they work? Best practice & research. *Clinical endocrinology & metabolism*. 2008 Oct;22(5):831–47.

[76] Fellner M, Baum RP, Kubícek V, Hermann P, Lukes I, Prasad V, et al. PET/CT imaging of osteoblastic bone metastases with (68)Ga-bisphosphonates: first human study. *European journal of nuclear medicine and molecular imaging*. 2010 Apr;37(4):834.

[77] Wang D, Sima M, Mosley RL, Davda JP, Tietze N, Miller C, et al. Pharmacokinetic and biodistribution studies of a bone-targeting drug delivery system based on N-(2-hydroxypropyl) methacrylamide copolymers. *Molecular Pharmaceutics*. 2006;3(6):717–25.

[78] Li J, Miller M a, Hutchins GD, Burr DB. Imaging bone microdamage in vivo with positron emission tomography. *Bone*. 2005 Dec;37(6):819–24.

[79] Srivastava P, Tiwari AK, Chadha N, Chuttani K, Mishra AK. Synthesis and biological evaluation of newly designed phosphonate based bone-

seeking agent. *European journal of medicinal chemistry*. 2013 Jul;65:12–20.

[80] Low S, Kopeček J. Targeting polymer therapeutics to bone. *Advanced drug delivery reviews*. 2012;64(12):1189–204.

[81] Weissleder R. Molecular Imaging: Exploring the Next Frontier. *Radiology*. 1999;212(3):609–14.

[82] Massoud TF, Gambhir SS. Molecular imaging in living subjects: seeing fundamental biological processes in a new light. *Genes & development*. 2003 Mar 1;17(5):545–80.

[83] Snoeks T, Khmelinskii A, Lelieveldt B. Optical advances in skeletal imaging applied to bone metastases. *Bone*. 2011;48(1):106–14.

[84] Zaheer a, Lenkinski RE, Mahmood a, Jones a G, Cantley LC, Frangioni J V. In vivo near-infrared fluorescence imaging of osteoblastic activity. *Nature biotechnology*. 2001 Dec;19(12):1148–54.

[85] Kozloff KM, Volakis LI, Marini JC, Caird MS. Near-infrared fluorescent probe traces bisphosphonate delivery and retention in vivo. *Journal of bone and mineral research*. 2010 Aug;25(8):1748–58.

[86] Kozloff KM, Weissleder R, Mahmood U. Noninvasive optical detection of bone mineral. *Journal of bone and mineral research*. 2007;22(8):1208–16.

[87] Gompels LL, Madden L, Lim NH, Inglis JJ, McConnell E, Vincent TL, et al. In vivo fluorescence imaging of E-selectin: quantitative detection of endothelial activation in a mouse model of arthritis. *Arthritis and rheumatism*. 2011 Jan;63(1):107–17.

[88] Lai W-FT, Chang C-H, Tang Y, Bronson R, Tung C-H. Early diagnosis of osteoarthritis using cathepsin B sensitive near-infrared fluorescent probes. *OsteoArthritis and Cartilage*. 2004 Mar;12(3):239–44.

[89] Ntziachristos V, Tung C-H, Bremer C, Weissleder R. Fluorescence molecular tomography resolves protease activity in vivo. *Nature medicine*. 2002 Jul;8(7):757–60.

[90] Kozloff KM, Quinti L, Patntirapong S, Hauschka P V, Tung C-H, Weissleder R, et al. Non-invasive optical detection of cathepsin K-mediated fluorescence reveals osteoclast activity in vitro and in vivo. *Bone*. 2009 Feb;44(2):190–8.

[91] Contag CH, Jenkins D, Contag PR, Negrin RS. Use of reporter genes for optical measurements of neoplastic disease in vivo. *Neoplasia*. 2000;2(1-2):41–52.

[92] Yang M, Baranov E, Jiang P, Sun FX, Li XM, Li L, et al. Whole-body optical imaging of green fluorescent protein-expressing tumors and

metastases. *Proceedings of the National Academy of Sciences of the United States of America*. 2000 Feb 1;97(3):1206–11.

[93] Wetterwald A, van der Pluijm G, Que I, Sijmons B, Buijs J, Karperien M, et al. Optical imaging of cancer metastasis to bone marrow: a mouse model of minimal residual disease. *The American journal of pathology*. 2002 Mar;160(3):1143–53.

[94] Corn DJ, Kim Y, Krebs MD, Mounts T, Molter J, Gerson S, et al. Imaging early stage osteogenic differentiation of mesenchymal stem cells. *Journal of orthopaedic research*. 2013 Jun;31(6):871–9.

[95] Marijanović I, Jiang X, Kronenberg MS, Stover ML, Erceg I, Lichtler AC, et al. Dual reporter transgene driven by 2.3Col1a1 promoter is active in differentiated osteoblasts. *Croatian medical journal*. 2003 Aug;44(4):412–7.

[96] Granero-Moltó F, Weis JA, Miga MI, Landis B, J.Myers T, O'Rear L, et al. Regenerative effects of transplanted mesenchymal stem cells in fracture healing. *Stem Cells*. 2009;27(8):1887–98.

[97] Iris B, Zilberman Y, Zeira E, Galun E, Honigman A, Turgeman G, et al. Molecular imaging of the skeleton: quantitative real-time bioluminescence monitoring gene expression in bone repair and development. *Journal of bone and mineral research*. 2003 Mar;18(3):570–8.

[98] Takahashi K, Onodera S, Tohyama H, Kwon HJ, Honma K, Yasuda K. In vivo imaging of particle-induced inflammation and osteolysis in the calvariae of NFκB/luciferase transgenic mice. *Journal of biomedicine & biotechnology*. 2011 Jan;2011.

[99] Ren P-G, Irani A, Huang Z, Ma T, Biswal S, Goodman SB. Continuous infusion of UHMWPE particles induces increased bone macrophages and osteolysis. *Clinical orthopaedics and related research*. 2011 Jan;469(1):113–22.

[100] Langton C, Palmer S, Porter R. The measurement of broadband ultrasonic attenuation in cancellous bone. *Engineering in medicine*. 1984;

[101] Langton CM, Njeh CF. The measurement of broadband ultrasonic attenuation in cancellous bone--a review of the science and technology. *IEEE transactions on ultrasonics, ferroelectrics, and frequency control*. 2008 Jul;55(7):1546–54.

[102] Rohrbach D, Preininger B, Hesse B, Gerigk H, Perka C, Raum K. The early phases of bone healing can be differentiated in a rat osteotomy

model by focused transverse-transmission ultrasound. *Ultrasound in medicine & biology*. 2013 Sep;39(9):1642–53.

[103] Fleming RH, Korver D, McCormack H a, Whitehead CC. Assessing bone mineral density in vivo: digitized fluoroscopy and ultrasound. *Poultry science*. 2004 Feb;83(2):207–14.

[104] Liukkonen J, Hirvasniemi J, Joukainen a, Penttilä P, Virén T, Saarakkala S, et al. Arthroscopic ultrasound technique for simultaneous quantitative assessment of articular cartilage and subchondral bone: an in vitro and in vivo feasibility study. *Ultrasound in medicine & biology*. 2013 Aug;39(8):1460–8.

[105] Klein MO, Grötz K a, Manefeld B, Kann PH, Al-Nawas B. Ultrasound transmission velocity for noninvasive evaluation of jaw bone quality in vivo before dental implantation. *Ultrasound in medicine & biology*. 2008 Dec;34(12):1966–71.

[106] Al-Nawas B, Klein MO, Götz H, Vaterod J, Duschner H, Grötz KA, et al. Dental implantation: ultrasound transmission velocity to evaluate critical bone quality--an animal model. Ultraschall in der Medizin. 2008 Jun 5;29(3):302–7.

[107] Kämmerer PW, Kumar V V, Brüllmann D, Götz H, Kann PH, Al-Nawas B, et al. Evaluation of ultrasound transmission velocity and 3-dimensional radiology in different bone types for dental implantology: a comparative ex vivo study. *Oral and Maxillofacial surgery*. 2013 Aug;116(2):e77–84.

[108] Mano I, Horii K, Matsukawa M, Otani T. Trial of Human Bone Cross-Sectional Imaging In vivo, Using Ultrasonic Echo Waves. *Japanese Journal of Applied* . 2013;52:5–7.

[109] Hangiandreou N. APM/RSNA physics tutorial for residents: Topics in US - B-mode US: Basic concepts and new technology. *Radiographics*. 2003;23(4):1019–33.

[110] Jaiswal RS, Singh J, Adams GP. High-resolution ultrasound biomicroscopy for monitoring ovarian structures in mice. *Reproductive biology and endocrinology*. 2009 Jan;7:69.

In: *In Vivo* Imaging: New Research
Editors: R. Hough and J. Camarillo
ISBN: 978-1-62948-633-8

Chapter 4

Manganese-Enhanced MRI: *In Vivo* Imaging of CNS Anatomy, Fiber Connectivity and Functional Activity

Ronny Haenold*
Leibniz Institute for Age Research,
Fritz Lipmann Institute e.V., Jena, Germany

Abstract

Imaging distinct neuronal networks and testing their functionality *in vivo* is challenging. While conventional magnetic resonance imaging (MRI) that is based on tissue-specific water relaxation provides detailed insight into the structural organization of the brain, manganese-enhanced MRI (MEMRI) affords additional layers of information regarding cellular composition, functional connectivity and activity within the CNS. Pioneered by A.P. Koretsky in 1998, it has emerged as a highly versatile and reliable tool for qualitative and quantitative neuroimaging. The expansion of MEMRI applications has been promoted by the increase in transgenic mouse models and the sophisticated technical progress achieved for small rodent MRI. The technique exploits the paramagnetic properties of manganese (Mn^{2+}), which augments MR contrast mainly by

* email: rhaenold@fli-leibniz.de.

shortening the T_1 spin-lattice relaxation time. As a calcium (Ca^{2+}) analog, it is incorporated into neurons by voltage-gated Ca^{2+} channels and actively transported along the axonal cytoskeleton. While Mn^{2+} accumulates in synaptic target areas, trans-synaptic propagation and re-uptake into secondary or tertiary neuronal circuits are limited. Thus, MEMRI represents a highly selective *in vivo* method for imaging brain anatomy, fiber connectivity, and neuronal activity with low unintentional background signaling. Mn^{2+} can be delivered by systemic administration for imaging neuroarchitectural features and mapping active brain areas or applied topically, e.g. via intranasal and intraocular microinjections to visualize primary sensory projections. In such studies, Mn^{2+}-dependent signal enhancement within axonal target regions represents a quantitative measure for structural integrity and metabolic viability of axonal connection, e.g. during post-traumatic de- and reorganization of axonal fibers and for assessing axonal transport impairments after genetic or pharmacological interventions. For each application, MEMRI protocols detailing optimized dose-responses for individual animal models are available, thus enabling repetitive and longitudinal *in vivo* studies without Mn^{2+} toxicity. Given the broad spectrum of MEMRI applications, this chapter serves as a useful and informative introduction for new users, but also will be of interest to more experienced operators. The chapter further discusses currently unresolved questions and future perspectives of MEMRI. For example, the observation that signal enhancement along the retino-tectal projection is unaffected in poor-sighted mice raises important questions about the electrophysiological properties that affect neuronal uptake and axonal transport of Mn^{2+}. Exciting technical modifications are presently underway that will further promote the applicability of MEMRI. One approach is working towards the precipitation of Mn^{2+} by autometallography to combine *in toto* MRI of CNS structures with the histological detection of Mn^{2+} at the cellular level. Other MEMRI studies have already demonstrated that Mn^{2+} toxicity can be reduced by topical delivery as eye drops or by safe circulatory release from Mn^{2+} derivatives. Thus, diagnostic applications to monitor cerebral functions and neuropathological alterations in humans are envisaged in the near future.

Introduction

General Considerations for *In Vivo* MRI

Of the various approaches for *in vivo* imaging of tissues, organs or complete organisms, magnetic resonance imaging (MRI) based on tissue-specific differences in proton relaxation time provides detailed anatomical information with high spatial resolution. In experimental MRI, the immobilized positioning of anesthetized animals allows for non-invasive imaging under almost physiological conditions, including repetitive recordings of individual subjects in longitudinal studies. MR images are generally of exquisite soft tissue contrast and are predestined for white and gray matter differentiation of the brain. Refinements in image acquisition and analysis additionally allow the correlation of molecular parameters, such as diffusion of water molecules (*diffusion MRI*) and cerebral blood flow (*functional MRI*) with neuroanatomical and neurophysiological properties, respectively. An example of diffusion MRI represents *diffusion tensor imaging* (DTI), which relies on the assessment of the spatial diffusion directions of water for imaging fiber connectivity [1]. Since the structural composition and organization of tissues affect the three-dimensional symmetry of water diffusion, highly myelinated structures such as tracts and nerves provide preferential diffusion parallel and restricted diffusion perpendicular to the tracts. The fiber direction is then calculated from the diffusion directions by post-processing algorithms. In clinical and experimental neuroimaging this application is termed tractography [2]. A disadvantage of diffusion MRI is its inability to discriminate between proximal-distal directions of identified axonal tracts and to assess their functional activity. Consequently, *blood oxygenation level-dependent* (BOLD) functional MRI is the method of choice to visualize local changes in neuronal activity during sensoric stimulation or cerebral processing [3]. BOLD enables live recordings of brain function by the detection of temporo-spatial changes in blood supply which emerge in regions of enhanced neuronal activity due to neurovascular coupling. While the obtained hemodynamic maps correlate well with brain activation, BOLD recordings do not provide direct information on neuronal activity, which is defined by electrical depolarization and induction of action potentials. Moreover, the detected activation patterns depend on the type and level of anesthesia, which therefore requires careful monitoring during contemporary stimulation and image acquisition [4]. For a variety of neurobiological studies, it would be highly desirable to achieve labeling of fiber connections or active brain areas under physiological conditions and defined environmental settings, and subsequently to record these patterns within short acquisition times. The combination of *in vivo* MRI with tracers that respond to neuronal physiology and activity would address such requirements. As a prototype, application of the divalent manganese ion (Mn^{2+}) has been employed as a contrast agent in manganese-enhanced MRI (MEMRI). MEMRI is a molecular imaging method for the visualization of neuronal connectivity and anatomy, as well as for brain activity *in vivo* [5]. As exemplified for the visual system, MEMRI bridges *in vivo* functional assays and *post-mortem* histology for the characterization of nerve fiber integrity under naïve and pathological conditions (Figure 1). While visually guided functional tasks, such as optometry or water maze, implicate complex sensomotoric processing and contain neurobehavioral components, characterization of the visual system by MEMRI provides unique insights into the activity of retinal layers and the retino-tectal fiber tract. Supplementary to histological sections and diffusion-weighted MRI to visualize the topographical projection of optic nerve fibers, MEMRI provides additional data on their neuroanatomy and viability. To date, MEMRI has been vigorously validated in more than 800 studies and usage of Mn^{2+} as an MRI contrast agent has become an invaluable tool in the field of neuroimaging today. Given the unique biophysical features of the manganese ion, the first part of the chapter covers general considerations for MEMRI. This is followed by a more detailed review of representative MEMRI studies on the rodent CNS.

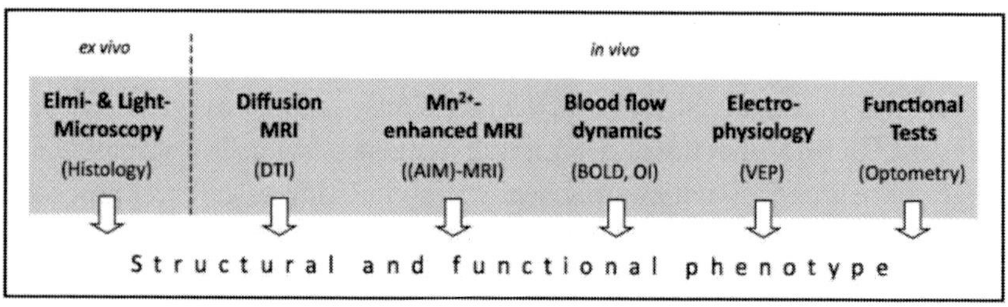

Figure 1. Integration of MEMRI into classical neurobiological methodology exemplified for studies on the visual system. Mn^{2+}-induced signal enhancement allows for qualitative and quantitative evaluation of phenotypes. Supplementary to histological sections and diffusion MRI (diffusion tensor imaging; DTI), the topographical projection of axonal fibers can be visualized by Mn^{2+} enhancement *in vivo*. When assigned as a Ca^{2+} analog, Mn^{2+}-induced signal enhancement in brain nuclei and nerve fiber projections can serve as a measure for the electrophysiological activity of neuronal circuits. Thereby, MEMRI provides direct information on neuronal activity, which supplements the elicitation of visual-evoked potentials (VEP) or visual tasks (optometry), and complements the assessment of hemodynamic changes in response to neurovascular coupling, e.g. by blood oxygenation level-dependent (BOLD) functional MRI or optical imaging (OI) of intrinsic signals. [Adopted and reproduced from [40]. Reprinted with the permission of Elsevier].

Biophysical Properties of Manganese

Manganese has an 80-year history as a biologically essential trace mineral [6, 7]. Chemically, it occurs in 11 different oxidation states (valences between –3 and +7), with the +2 valence being the most prevalent ionic state in biological tissues. Mn^{2+} acts as a cofactor to catalyze enzymatic reactions and to modulate binding specificities of surface receptors and extracellular matrix proteins. The classes of enzymes and metallo-proteins that incorporate Mn^{2+} are very broad and, thus, highlight the essentiality of Mn^{2+} for cell biology. Without any claim to completeness, this list includes manganese superoxide dismutase, pyruvate carboxylase, glutamine synthetase, galactosyltransferase, arginase, lyases, isomerases, ligases, as well as integrins and lectins [8]. The physiological tissue concentration of Mn^{2+} varies between 3 and 20 μM in adult organisms, although maximum levels of 200 μM and higher have been detected in some brain areas of rats [9]. The major source of Mn^{2+} is food intake and dedicated mechanisms for nutritional absorption, transport in blood and visceral fluids, uptake into tissues and cells, intracellular storage, and hepatic elimination of the ion exist [10, 11]. For MEMRI applications, it is elementary that cellular uptake of manganese ions is linked to iron (Fe) and, most relevant, to calcium (Ca^{2+}) homeostasis [8]. Mn^{3+} present in the extracellular space competes for the Fe^{3+}-binding protein transferrin. It is transported as a transferrin complex within the circulatory system and becomes readily internalized through cell membranes via transferrin receptor-mediated endocytosis. Intracellular uptake of Mn^{2+} can be mediated by the divalent metal transporter 1. However, the physiological role for entry of Mn^{2+} into the cerebral endothelium and for passing the blood-brain barrier by this mechanism is under debate [12]. Notably, the Mn^{2+} ion passes through voltage- and ligand-gated Ca^{2+} channels [13, 14]. The rationale for the occupation of Ca^{2+} channels by Mn^{2+} is the identical electric charge and the similar ionic radius of both ions (Mn^{2+}: 91 pm; Ca^{2+}: 106 pm). Given the high relevance of Ca^{2+} as a second messenger in neuronal tissue, channel-mediated influx is assumed to be the dominant mechanism for intracellular uptake of Mn^{2+} in the CNS [13, 14]. Since opening of voltage-gated Ca^{2+} channels is a hallmark of neuronal excitability, significant amounts of Mn^{2+} can enter neurons, particularly during depolarization. Early studies that utilized the radioactive isotope ^{54}Mn monitored the electrophysiological properties of Mn^{2+} uptake. Thereby, they compared the time courses for the voltage-dependent influx of the two ions into synaptosomes prepared from the rat CNS [15]. The kinetics of intracellular Mn^{2+} uptake after membrane depolarization by K^+ is characterized by an initially high transition rate, which gradually levels off within 10 seconds. Such kinetics is typical for influx through both fast inactivating and slow non-inactivating Ca^{2+} channels. While the overall permeability rate of Mn^{2+} is about 2.6-fold lower compared to Ca^{2+} [15], glutamate receptor stimulation further enhances Mn^{2+} uptake [16]. Conversely, entry into cells is inhibited by diverse Ca^{2+} channel blockers such as verapamil. These inhibitors can block the influx of Mn^{2+} even more effectively than that of Ca^{2+} [15].

In contrast to the similar properties for uptake of Mn^{2+} and Ca^{2+} from extracellular media, the efflux out of synaptosomes is strikingly different for these two ions [15]. Release of Ca^{2+} back into the medium is readily stimulated by a depolarizing solution containing K^+ and Na^+, whereas active segregation of Mn^{2+} from synaptosomes is not detectable. Although not yet fully understood, one reason might be that intracellular proteins comprehensively sequester the Mn^{2+} ion. As initially suggested from isolated synaptosomes, *in vivo* accumulation of Mn^{2+} within the neuronal compartment could be confirmed by both clinical and experimental studies that investigated the biodistribution of Mn^{2+} within challenged animals and exposed patients [17-19]. Thus, ready uptake into excitable cells via Ca^{2+} channels in combination with its negligible extracellular release results in a long retention time for Mn^{2+} within neuronal cells. These early studies on cellular Mn^{2+} turnover are elementary for its correct application as an anatomic and functional tracer in MEMRI (Figure 2). Thereby, the following properties require specific considerations for setting up MEMRI experiments. First, Mn^{2+} acts as an intracellular MRI contrast agent, thus Mn^{2+}-enhanced anatomical structures are of cellular origin. Such a property is different from other contrast agents, such as systemically applied gadolinium which provides tissue contrast by vascular and interstitial enhancement. While the latter substance is superior at detecting anomalies in the neurovascular system, such as clogging of blood vessels or disruption of the blood-brain barrier, it does not detail immediate information on the neuroarchitecture or activity. Secondly, the velocity of Mn^{2+} uptake, intracellular distribution, and retention define the kinetics and clearance time for MEMRI signal enhancement. After influx through Ca^{2+} channels, Mn^{2+} accumulates in the cytoplasm due to protein binding or storage within vesicles. It becomes intracellularly distributed along axonal processes by fast axonal transport. Thus, the optimal time point for image acquisition of the fully established contrast pattern requires a post-application latency phase of several hours, as will be discussed later. Due to the long half-life of Mn^{2+} in neuronal tissue compared to its short half-life in visceral organs like the heart and liver, signal enhancement in the brain lasts for several days. Practically, this feature is useful to cumulatively increase the intracerebral Mn^{2+} concentration and to boost MEMRI contrast by fractionated injections of low-toxicity dosages (i.e. 30 mg/kg body weight) systematically delivered at 48-hr intervals [20]. Finally, complex formation with intracellular proteins limits the histological detectability of Mn^{2+}, i.e. using commonly applied silver precipitation techniques (autometallography) [21]. Since this method relies on the presence of free metal ions, a majority of Mn^{2+} bound to proteins remains undetectable so far [22].

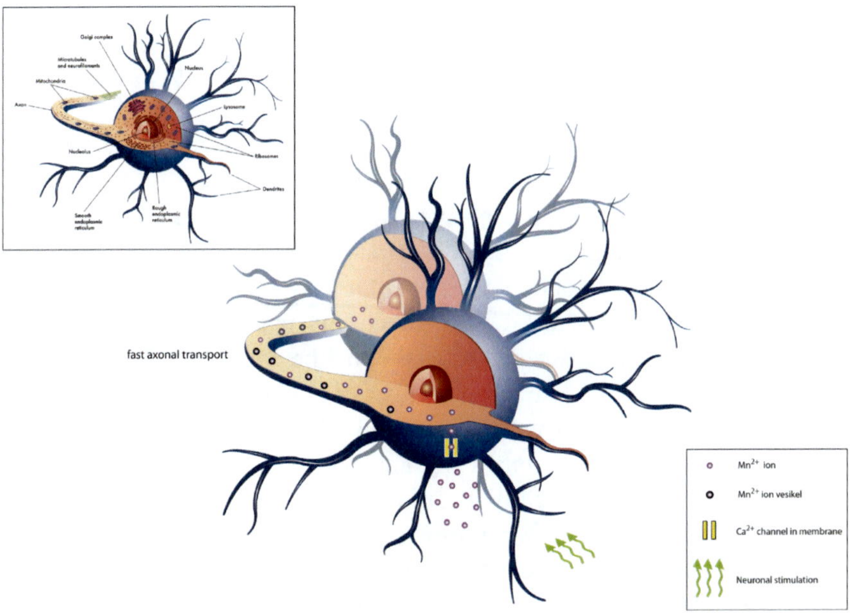

Figure 2. Schematic illustration of neuronal Mn^{2+} uptake and axonal propagation. Systemically or topically applied Mn^{2+} enters excitable neurons predominantly via Ca^{2+} channels to become intracellularly accumulated within the cytosolic and vesicular compartments. Fast axonal transport, together with limited trans-synaptic propagation are the origin for its specific distribution within CNS neuronal circuits, e.g. the retino-tectal or cortico-thalamic projection. MEMRI signal intensity in cerebral nuclei and along fiber tracts depends on various physiological parameters, including local Mn^{2+} dosage and neurotoxicity, neuronal density and activity, as well as axonal integrity.

As a Ca^{2+} analog, Mn^{2+} interferes with Ca^{2+}-dependent physiological processes by multiple ways, a fact that should be considered for the experimental administration of Mn^{2+} in MEMRI. Since both ions compete for the same channels, Mn^{2+} is a competitive inhibitor of Ca^{2+} influx. Increased

Mn^{2+} influx due to elevated extracellular Mn^{2+} concentrations reduces voltage-dependent Ca^{2+} uptake, which might affect neuronal Ca^{2+} metabolism. Moreover, Mn^{2+} shares a number of transport mechanisms for iron and copper. It is conceivable that high levels of Mn^{2+} compete with their transport pathways and for occupation to regulatory proteins, leading to a decreased uptake of these metals in brain. Indeed, the concentration of iron is significantly reduced in the thalamus of mice that received four Mn^{2+} dosages of 30 mg/kg body weight [23]. Likewise, levels of iron and zinc within the hippocampal CA3/dentate gyrus areas are significantly decreased to 56.6% and 73.6%, respectively, following intraperitoneal or intracerebral Mn^{2+} applications [24]. Putative bystander effects on MR relaxation of brain tissue that are associated with altered metal homeostasis by Mn^{2+} have not yet been investigated.

Similar to Ca^{2+}, Mn^{2+} triggers the release of various neurotransmitters, such as dopamine, 5-hydroxy tyrosine or γ-aminobutyric acid (GABA), from synaptosomes that are incubated in a depolarizing K^+-rich solution. This effect is observed for concentrations as low as 1 mM Mn^{2+}, although the amount of segregated transmitter is about 6-fold lower for Mn^{2+} compared to Ca^{2+}. When both ions are co-administered, the effect on transmitter release is not synergistic, suggesting that Mn^{2+} acts on the regular Ca^{2+}-dependent transmitter pool. Such a transmitter-releasing potential of Mn^{2+} might contribute to the clinical symptoms observed after Mn^{2+} intoxication. It also may have relevance for the animal's physiology in MEMRI experiments.

The preferential accessibility of the brain for Mn^{2+} is long known from studies on ^{54}Mn-treated rats and primates [17, 25], and goes back further to metal workers and miners that suffered from health impairments after chronic exposure to Mn^{2+}-enriched fumes. The neurological deficits observed after systemic intoxication with Mn^{2+} resemble those of Parkinson's disease and are clinically defined as Manganism [26, 27]. Fundamental to the high neurotoxic potential of Mn^{2+} are the versatile entrance routes into the CNS and the affinity of brain tissue for Mn^{2+} accumulation. Systemically injected Mn^{2+} readily enters the brain via two routes, the blood-brain barrier and the blood-cerebrospinal fluid choroid plexus, from where it is further distributed into the tissue. After systemic delivery, either by intravenous or subcutaneous injections into humans and non-human primates, the half-life of elimination from the CNS is about 50 days [18, 28]. When Mn^{2+} is inhaled, this time is extended to 260 days. Such delayed elimination from the CNS is due to continuous circulatory replenishment of originally deposited Mn^{2+} from the lungs [18]. Additionally, inhaled Mn^{2+} is taken up from the nasal epithelium to directly enter the brain via olfactory and trigeminal nerves [29].

Within the organism, Mn^{2+} is predominantly metabolized in liver and kidney. In the brain, astrocytes are a major reservoir for endogenous Mn^{2+}, where it is bound to the enzyme glutamine synthetase to foster enzymatic activity. Such protein binding is considered as an effective buffer system to keep free Mn^{2+} concentrations to physiological levels [30]. It also may be involved in the detoxification of excessively applied Mn^{2+} [31], such as in MEMRI studies. Indeed, the hyperintensive signal in the hippocampal fissure, which is mainly composed of astrocytes and is visible after Mn^{2+} administration, might originate from astroglia-mediated buffering of Mn^{2+} [24]. However, it is still difficult to ascertain the exact cellular targets of Mn^{2+} in the hippocampal fissure on the meso-scale level of MEMRI. In general, it is well accepted that neurons are the primary target of supplementary applied Mn^{2+}. This finding has emerged from early biochemical studies. ^{54}Mn topically injected into the rat striatum or substantia nigra is taken up by striatal and nigral neurons to get transported along the striatonigral and nigrostriatal projections, as detected by autoradiography of dissected brain tissue. Notably, unilateral colchicine injection or transection of the median forebrain bundle abolishes the distribution along fiber connections and accumulation in projection-specific target regions [32, 33]. These early radiographic observations reflect many of the properties of Mn^{2+} as a molecular tracer that have subsequently been observed by *in vivo* MEMRI. The circuitry-specific distribution of Mn^{2+} points to a limited trans-synaptic propagation. Although not yet fully understood, data from the visual system indicate that synaptic release and uptake of Mn^{2+} by post-synaptic neurons is linked to neuronal depolarization and requires the formation of action potentials [34]. The presence of Mn^{2+} within synaptic vesicles is shown, at least, for glutamatergic neurons. Thus, it is assumed that vesicular Mn^{2+} may be concurrently released with the stimulatory neurotransmitter glutamate [35].

Manganese is detectable by MRI due to the paramagnetic properties of its ionic states. Causative for the paramagnetism is the presence of unpaired electrons, which endues the ion with a strong magnetic momentum. For example, in the +2 oxidation state of Mn^{2+}, the paramagnetism originates from the removal of the two outermost 4s electrons. This leaves its 3d orbitals half occupied by five single electrons. The magnetic field arising from the paramagnetic manganese ion causes local fluctuations and, thereby, causes a shortening of the spin-lattice relaxation time T_1 of surrounding water protons. This difference in the relaxation time is the reason that Mn^{2+} can be used as a contrast agent in T_1-weighted MRI. In principle, it is likewise possible to choose T_2 weighting (spin-spin relaxation time) for MEMRI. Under practical considerations, T_1-based weighting is the option of choice for *in vivo* imaging because it increases the Mn^{2+}-dependent signal intensity and thereby provides a positive ('bright') contrast enhancement of the tissue.

With respect to Mn^{2+}-dependent contrast enhancement in biological tissues, MEMRI only detects Mn^{2+} and Mn^{3+}, but it is insensitive towards elementary manganese. Binding of Mn^{2+} to intracellular proteins can alter the Mn^{2+} relaxation time in tissue compared to the paramagnetic properties of a pure Mn^{2+} solution. Such interaction may enhance MR sensitivity of Mn^{2+}, as previously described for albumin-bound gadolinium [36], but the exact mechanisms are not clearly defined [37, 38]. In general, there is a proportional relationship between the relaxation rate of water and the concentration of Mn^{2+}, resulting in decreased or increased contrasts for T_1 and T_2, respectively. Quantitatively, the pre-Mn^{2+} T_1 value in the murine hippocampus is 1,710±18.2 ms when measured at 11.7 T. It becomes shortened to 851.6±6.3 ms and 474.7±3.7 ms at around 24 hr after infusion of 44 mg/kg body weight Mn^{2+} and 175 mg/kg body weight Mn^{2+}, respectively. In the pituitary gland, which shows the strongest accumulation of Mn^{2+} among all brain areas, T_1 becomes even more shortened from 1,167±25.7 ms to 142.6±42.8 ms at the highest Mn^{2+} dosage [39]. To make use of the reduced relaxation times in T_1-weighted MEMRI, established protocols are available. They routinely enable imaging at an isotropic resolution below $(200\ \mu m)^3$ with relatively short recording times of about 30 to 90 min [40]. However, the respective scan parameters applied depend on the individual scanner and coil specificities, as well as on the specific demand for image acquisition that is best suited to answer the individual scientific question.

Manganese-Enhanced Magnetic Resonance Imaging (MEMRI)

The concept that soluble Mn^{2+} ions increase MRI signal intensity was introduced 30 years ago by P.C. Lauterbur when he discovered that addition of $MnSO_4$ shortens the relaxation time T_1 of a water sample [41]. M.H. Mendonça-Dias and her colleagues were the first to employ the paramagnetic properties of Mn^{2+} ions to alter the MRI contrast of extracted visceral organs, whereby they localized ischemic areas [42]. These studies are elementary for the subsequent evolution of MEMRI because they demonstrate the proof-of-principle that Mn^{2+} supplementation provides selective MRI contrast in biological tissues. Consequently, MRI was applied thereafter to detect Mn^{2+} accumulation in the basal ganglia of primates that were poisoned by inhalation or intravenous application of $MnCl_2$ [43]. The evident loco-temporal distribution of Mn^{2+} within distinct parts of the nervous system correlated well with the prototypical functional impairments observed for Manganism, thus revealing the feasibility of MEMRI as a diagnostic tool for Mn^{2+} intoxication. While the authors at the same time recognized the potential of Mn^{2+} as a contrast agent, they questioned its applicability in clinical and experimental studies due to its neurotoxicity. Today, A.P. Koretsky and colleagues are recognized as the founders of applied MEMRI and without doubt the technique was pioneered by their groundbreaking studies on rodents [37, 44-46]. Highly illuminative of the outstanding progression of MEMRI is the fact that mice were killed before the scan in early studies because of the initially long acquisition time of 2.7 hr [45]. Since then, the technique has been systematically refined for applications in different animals, including the sea snail, crayfish, fish, amphibians, songbirds, rabbits, and non-human primates, where it is utilized for imaging of the nervous system, liver, heart, colon or pancreas. Given the rich biology of Mn^{2+} and the particularly high affinity of Mn^{2+} for neuronal cells [24], the method has evolved from steady-state imaging of neuronal anatomy towards longitudinal assessments of highly dynamic processes, such as neuronal activity and axonal transport, as well as structural plasticity, injury, and repair. While serial scans following a single Mn^{2+} application allow for kinetic estimations of Mn^{2+} distribution, plastic changes of the neuronal network can be followed over time by repetitive imaging of individual specimens. The high versatility of MEMRI also emanates from the simplicity of the tracer which is administered as a conveniently available $MnCl_2$ solution and from the different delivery routes by which Mn^{2+} can be applied. For systemic enhancement of the rodent brain, intraperitoneal, intravenous, subcutaneous or intramuscular Mn^{2+} injections at dosages of 44 mg/kg body weight (rat) and up to 66 mg/kg body weight (mouse) are feasible [47]. Alternatively, Mn^{2+} can be directly applied to target cell populations for region-specific uptake, e.g. after intranasal, intraretinal or intracerebral loadings at concentrations of 10–100 mM Mn^{2+}. The rationale for all applications is the assumption that MEMRI signal enhancement correlates with the local Mn^{2+} concentration. Recently, a quantitative study measured the Mn^{2+} concentrations in the hippocampus after intraperitoneal Mn^{2+} injection by MEMRI and X-ray fluorescence (SR-XRF) microprobing. The study shows a good correlation between the increase in MEMRI signal intensity (T_1-weighted signal-to-noise ratio: +81%) and manganese concentrations determined by SR-XRF ([Mn]: +100%; r^2=0.93; p<0.002) [24]. Such a linear increase in T_1-weighted signal enhancement is crucial for performing quantitative MEMRI analyses and for comparing Mn^{2+} accumulation under various experimental conditions. In the following section, the three main applications for MEMRI, (i) neural architecture [48], (ii) neuronal connections [45], and (iii) neuronal activation [44], are presented. Given the increasingly high number of publications on MEMRI, the selected examples are far from being complete. However, they have been chosen to illustrate the broad applicability of MEMRI for modern neuroimaging.

Anatomy and Neuroarchitecture

The applicability of MEMRI to enhance brain anatomy goes back to neurotoxicological studies that utilized MRI for mapping early ventricular uptake and subsequent intracerebral distribution of Mn^{2+} in rats and monkeys, respectively [43, 49]. These studies show that Mn^{2+} enters the brain through the choroid plexus to become accumulated in the gray matter, thus delineating the cerebral structure in a unique manner. Without contrast agents, the brain shows only weak tissue contrast in T_1-weighted images. Following systemic (intravenous, intraperitoneal, intramuscular or subcutaneous) application, Mn^{2+} gains its function as a whole-brain contrast agent by preferential and gradual accumulation in neuronal somata. Depending on the cellular density and the rate of Mn^{2+} uptake, different neuronal nuclei and laminar structures are clearly discernible from ventricles and axonal fiber tracts. The enhancement is optimally imaged at about 24 hr after injection, when the heterogeneous enhancement pattern has finally evolved. Spatial enhancement of the brain follows a time-course that is determined by the fast (within minutes) uptake of Mn^{2+} from cerebral blood through the choroid plexus into ventricles and cerebrospinal fluid spaces. From there, it is distributed around the periventricular tissue zone and finally accumulates in neuronal target areas [39, 48, 50]. At this time point, clearance of Mn^{2+} from ventricles has already finished. Brain areas that are devoid of the blood-brain barrier, such as the pituitary gland and pineal gland, show an extraordinary rapid and strong signal increase. Figure 3 shows horizontal (left), sagittal (center), and axial (right) cuts from a typical T_1-weighted spin-echo 3D MRI of a mouse brain acquired 24 hr after intravenous infusion of increasing doses of Mn^{2+} [39]. At this time point, sections show additional enhancement of the CA1, CA2, CA3, and fimbria regions of the hippocampus, the arrowhead of the dentate gyrus, habenula, olfactory bulb, cerebellum, inferior colliculus, and interpeduncular nucleus (Figure 3).

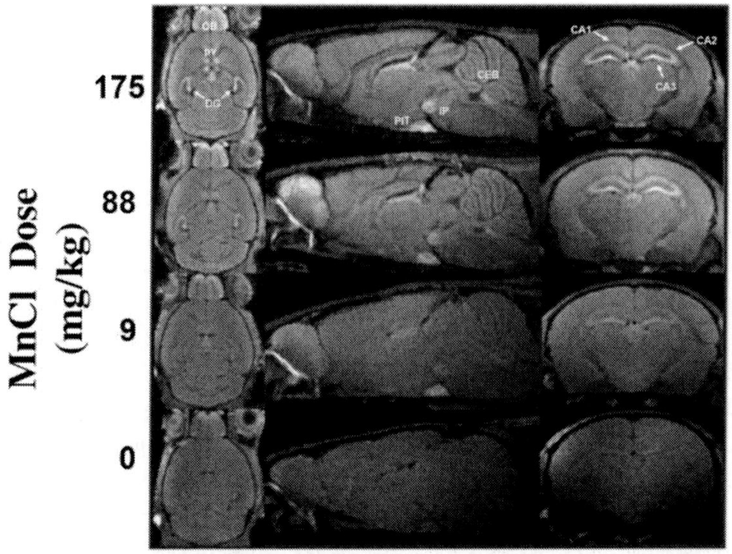

Figure 3. MEMRI for neuroarchitecture/anatomy. Dose dependence of MEMRI contrast. Typical horizontal (left), sagittal (center), and axial (right) cuts from representative T_1-weighted spin-echo 3D MEMRI of a mouse brain acquired 24 hr after systemic injection of varying doses of $MnCl_2$ are shown in each row. Enhancement of the brain is clearly visible even at the lowest dose of $MnCl_2$, especially in areas of the brain devoid of the blood-brain barrier, such as the pituitary and pineal glands, in periventricular zones, and in the olfactory bulb. Tissue-specific contrast enhancement progresses with increasing doses of $MnCl_2$, allowing for better delineation of subregional anatomic features, particularly within the hippocampus, olfactory bulb, cortex, and deep brain nuclei. CEB: cerebellum; CA1, CA2, CA3: CA formation of hippocampus; DG: dentate gyrus; IP: interpeduncular nucleus; OB: olfactory bulb; Pit: pituitary gland; pv: periventricular tissue zone. [Adopted and reproduced from [39]. Reprinted with the permission of Wiley-Liss, Inc., a subsidiary of John Wiley & Sons, Inc.].

Notably, the pattern of regional brain enhancement and intensity is typical yet not identical within all species, as demonstrated by species-specific differences for the murine and primate brain. For example, the striatum, which appears strongly enhanced in human patients and in marmosets after Mn^{2+} overexposure, is less pronounced in the rodent brain, as are the thalamus and visual cortex (V1) [51]. Besides differences in the brain uptake of Mn^{2+}, this might be related to different neuroanatomical features, i.e. the specific geometry of the lateral ventricles and third ventricle in primates which allows efficient propagation of Mn^{2+} into the neighboring striatum. Given the high affinity of the olfactory bulb for Mn^{2+} uptake, separate layers, such as the glomerular and mitral cell layers, are already clearly discernible at low dosages of 9 mg/kg body weight. High dosages of up to 175 mg/kg body weight allow for an excellent delineation of sub-regional anatomical features, such as the CA1, CA2, CA3, and fimbria regions within the hippocampus, cortical layers (IV), and the gray matter of the cerebellum [39]. As mentioned above, Mn^{2+} retains in the brain with only slow elimination within two weeks or more back to background signal intensities. Such a long half-life within the CNS can be used to circumvent the immediate toxicity caused by a single application of high Mn^{2+} dosages. In a previous study, excellent contrast enhancement of all the aforementioned brain areas is achieved by administration of six dosages of 30 mg/kg body weight each, applied every 48 hr. Such cumulative Mn^{2+} injections readily build up detectable doses in the brain, and tolerance is demonstrated by rats even over 12 injections [20].

The heterogeneous yet typical distribution of Mn^{2+} throughout the brain is highly useful to study brain abnormalities, especially in genetically altered mice. Given the advances in the field of mouse genetics and the increasing availability of mutants resembling human neurodevelopmental defects, the manifestation of such phenotypes can be optimally monitored by longitudinal MEMRI analysis of individual subjects. Thereby, utilization of MEMRI is not age-restricted to juvenile or adult animals. To monitor neurodevelopmental defects that often emerge during embryonic or early post-natal stages, Mn^{2+} can be readily delivered to pups by lactation following maternal injection. Such an administration regime was recently applied to validate the variable malformation of the vermis region, the central region of the cerebellum, in *gastrulation brain homeobox 2* (*Gbx2*) conditional *knockout* mice [52]. To enhance the foliated pattern of the cerebellum together with the deep cerebellar nuclei in a litter of newborn pups, the mother received intraperitoneal injections of an $MnCl_2$ solution at a common dosage of 80 mg/kg body weight. In each mouse, formation of the complex 3D structure of the cerebellar foliation was followed over time by repetitive scans, and graduated phenotypes associated with the loss of *Gbx2* can be dissected ranging from mild to severe cerebellar disorganization. Moreover, 3D renderings of the Mn^{2+}-enhanced cerebellar nuclei reveal altered shape and position in the *knockout*, an observation that can be easily missed by non-enhanced MRI [52]. Taken together, anatomical phenotypes and their temporal manifestation, as observed in the *Gbx2 knockout* mouse, are best appreciated using 3D MEMRI which is superior in detailing spatial and volumetric information on distinct brain structures compared to conventional MRI or histology.

The signal enhancement facilitated by Mn^{2+} within the cellular gray matter can be exploited to improve imaging of the myelin-rich white matter by enhancing white-gray matter contrast. Conventionally, myelinated structures such as nerves and fiber tracts are visualized using magnetization transfer (MT)-MRI that relies upon the indirect saturation of mobile water protons by intermittent (off-resonance) application of magnetization impulses. Since the protons in the lipid-rich myelin are bound to macromolecules, they are highly immobilized compared to the relatively free movement of protons in the gray matter or ventricular space. Thus, off-resonance polarization by magnetization impulses is significantly diminished and the fiber tracts appear with low intensity in MT-MR images. The contrasting effect of MT impulses should become further enhanced by accumulation of Mn^{2+} within non-white matter tissues. This paradigm was principally proven in a study by Watanabe and colleagues which aimed to improve myelin mapping in living mice [53, 54]. Thereby, Mn^{2+}-enhanced MT-MRI enables the identification of even small myelin-rich structures, such as the fornix, optic tract, stria medullaris of the thalamus, and mammillothalamic tract. As outlined above, these structures appear dark in signal intensity due to the T_1 weighting. Given the high number of clinical neuropathies that involve white matter distortions, this approach is expected to contribute to a better neuroanatomical characterization of animal models of human diseases, most notably experimental autoimmune encephalomyelitis.

Tract Tracing

After uptake by voltage-gated ion channels, Mn^{2+} accumulates in neuronal cell bodies and becomes distributed within the cytoplasmic compartment including axonal processes (Figure 2). The fact that Mn^{2+} moves along neuronal fiber pathways is a very useful property for MEMRI applications in neuronal tract tracing. Direction and speed of tracing are determined by (i) the anterograde fast axonal transport rate of around 2–3 mm/hr, depending on the investigated species and neuronal pathway [45, 55, 56]; (ii) the requirement of an active and microtubule-based transport machinery, as indicated by the fact that Mn^{2+} is preferentially accumulated in the microsomal fraction and its transport is blocked by colchicine [45, 57]; (iii) the saturated axonal transport and trans-synaptic propagation of Mn^{2+}, whereas passive diffusion or leakage from the cell is low [58]. These characteristics emerged from early studies on cerebral ^{54}Mn microinjections that showed region-specific distribution of the isotope along striatonigral fibers 4 hr after injection into the striatum. Transection of the medial forebrain bundle disrupted ^{54}Mn transport through these fibers and subsequently its accumulation within the substantia nigra [33, 57]. The identification and imaging of brain connectivity on the macroscopic scale by MEMRI appears as an immediate area of application for tract tracing, provided that Mn^{2+} can be stereotaxically injected to presynaptic neurons that form the respective projections. Indeed, the course of several pathways has been impressively illustrated by *in vivo* MEMRI, including ascending sensory and intracerebral trajectories. Given the good accessibility of the rodent eye and nostril for topical Mn^{2+} administration, primary visual and olfactory projections have been visualized first [45]. Meanwhile, numerous studies have optimized the technique with respect to the kinetics and toxicity of Mn^{2+}, particularly for uptake and transport along the visual system [59-61]. Following injection of a small volume into the vitreous body, Mn^{2+} is taken up by retinal ganglion cells (RGCs) and becomes transported along the optic nerve and optic tract up to the thalamic lateral geniculate nucleus (LGN) and subcortical superior colliculus (SC). A sagittal view on a rendered, 3D maximum intensity projection of the contrast-enhanced retino-tectal projection, imaged 24 hr after bilateral intravitreal injection of 15 nmol $MnCl_2$, is presented in Figure 4 [61]. Note the lack of significant trans-synaptic tracer propagation into visual cortical areas, which has been reported for more latent acquisition time points [62]. Visualization of the thalamo-cortical (LGN to primary visual cortex V1) and intracortical (V1 to contralateral V1/2 via visual callosal pathway) sections of the visual projection can be achieved by stage-wise tracing via subcortical (LGN) and intracortical (V1) injections [62].

Because Mn^{2+} propagation depends on cellular viability and the presence of intact axonal connections, its transport is impaired under chronic neurodegeneration and interrupted after traumatic nerve injury. Consequently, Mn^{2+}-dependent signal enhancement within the axonal projection area correlates with the overall number and viability of the tract-forming fibers and can be used to quantitatively assess axonal transport processes. To date, two main applications of tract tracing by MEMRI have proved highly valuable to characterize axonal neuropathologies in translational animal models. First, MEMRI is an excellent method to monitor temporo-spatial changes in response to acute nerve injury. The favored model to study axonal regeneration in the CNS is optic nerve crush injury. While intravitreal application of Mn^{2+} readily traces the retino-tectal projection up to the SC, Mn^{2+} propagation is abruptly stopped at the proximal stump of the injured optic nerve. Thus, MEMRI enables diagnostics of lesion sites with high spatial resolution [40]. Moreover, when the injury is incompletely inflicted in terms of anterior, posterior or lateral hemisection, only spared axon bundles reach their ancestral target areas within the SC. The pattern of such retinotopic target innervation has recently been precisely mapped by MEMRI [63].

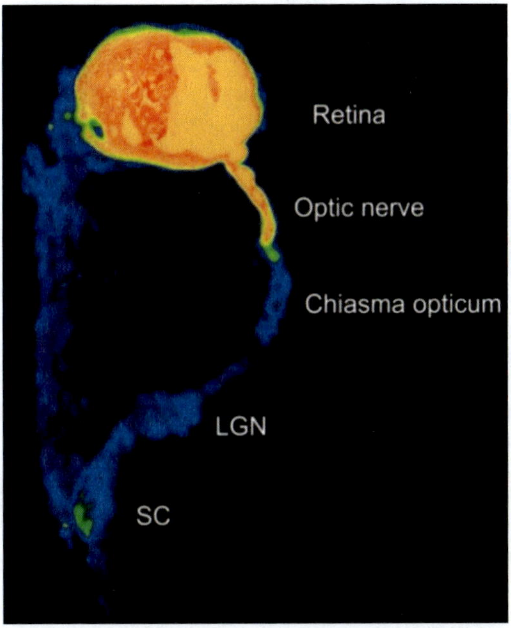

Figure 4. MEMRI of mouse visual projection. Sagittal view on a rendered 3D (maximum projection intensity) heat map presentation of the *in situ* contrast-enhanced retino-tectal projection. MRI was performed 24 hr after bilateral intravitreal injection of 15 nmol $MnCl_2$. [Adopted and reproduced from [61]. Reprinted with the permission of the *Journal of Visualized Experiments*].

Optic nerve injury is a commonly used model to study axonal regeneration in response to growth stimulatory treatments. Given the high demand to screen drugs and molecular biological interventions for their anti-apoptotic and pro-regenerative potentials, such treatment regimes could be readily validated in longitudinal studies using MEMRI. Initial attempts using intraretinal implantations of peripheral nerve grafts or olfactory ensheathing cell grafts are promising examples that MEMRI is suitable to monitor plastic changes within axonal lesion sites by repetitive MR scans [64, 65]. Currently, attempts to further improve the applicability of the tracer are under investigation, e.g. by topical loading as eye drops. While repeated loads of the Mn^{2+} solution on the cornea sufficiently enhance the retinal layers, further refinements are necessary to achieve substantial enhancement of the optic nerve [66]. Then, it is likely that tract-specific MEMRI could become a diagnostic tool for the broad range of retinopathies and other neuropathies.

The other application of tract-specific MEMRI is quantitative assessment of axonal transport processes, which is generally a challenging task in the living brain independent of the application of either MRI contrast agents or fluorescent tracers in microscopy. This is due, in particular, to the relative inaccessibility of appropriate neuronal tracts. For example, selective tracing of corticofugal somatosensory or motor pathways requires stereotaxic intracortical injections which need to be optimized to avoid negative side effects on tracer uptake and propagation due to tissue damage [31]. Minimal or even non-invasive application routes are intravitreal, intracochlear or intranasal administration to image primary visual, acoustic or olfactory fiber tracts, respectively. MEMRI is particularly sensitive in detecting subtle impairments in the axonal transport velocity of these fibers. As a consequence, quantitative MEMRI is established as a routine application to estimate transport perturbations in translational models of neuropathological diseases. First indications came from aging studies on rats that received small volumes of Mn^{2+} loaded into the nostrils, with results confirming the uptake of Mn^{2+} by primary neurons in the olfactory epithelium and its transport along the olfactory nerve into the olfactory bulb, and from there into the anterior olfactory nucleus and piriform nucleus of the cortex [67]. However, upon comparison of the time course of peak signal enhancement along the olfactory tract, the authors detected that bulk transport of Mn^{2+} is slowed by 58% in mid-age (13–17 months old) and up to 71% in old (24–25 months old) rats [67]. Subsequently, the system has been utilized to monitor early and progressive impairments in axonal transport rates in mouse models of Alzheimer's disease [68-70]. Such global analysis of axonal transport kinetics on the macroscopic scale of fiber tracts is enormously valuable to visualize the early changes in Alzheimer's disease brains and to facilitate the selection of neuroprotective drugs in preclinical trials.

Neuronal Activity

As outlined earlier, there is a preference for Mn^{2+} uptake by neurons through voltage-gated Ca^{2+} channels. Since Ca^{2+} influx is a hallmark of cellular excitability and Mn^{2+} can be considered as a quantitative surrogate for intracellular Ca^{2+} levels, Mn^{2+}-dependent MRI signal enhancement serves as a good correlate for neuronal activity. Thus, MEMRI can be employed – besides for the imaging of neuroanatomical structures – to map regional brain activity in response to neuronal stimulation. Such a functional MRI application using Mn^{2+} is referred to in the literature as activity-induced Mn^{2+}-dependent MRI (AIM-MRI). Conceptionally, it goes back to pioneering studies by Y.J. Lin and A.P. Koretsky (1997) showing that activation of the rat brain by injection of the excitatory transmitter glutamate increases MEMRI signal intensity to about 240% of the original [44]. In contrast to conventional functional MRI techniques that rely on detecting changes in hemodynamics, such as BOLD and cerebral blood flow, Ca^{2+}-dependent AIM-MRI enables imaging of a parameter that is directly related to neuronal activity. Notably, in a rat model of sensory forepaw stimulation, the MEMRI signal is specifically enhanced in the contralateral somatosensory cortex and the activation map overlaps quantitatively and spatially with co-registered BOLD and cerebral blood flow recordings [71]. Such studies impressively confirm the specificity and sensitivity of AIM-MRI towards changes in neuronal activation patterns, thus presenting exciting options for monitoring brain functions *in vivo*. To date, it has been utilized for tonotopic mapping of the rat inferior colliculus after acoustic stimulation with noise bursts ranging in frequency from 25 to 65 kHz [72, 73]. Thereby, the auditory network including the accessory structures cochlear nucleus, lateral lemniscus, and superior olivary complex are enhanced in exposed rats compared to animals housed in a quiet environment [73]. Intratympanic Mn^{2+} administration has revealed sound intensity- and frequency-dependent functional activity in the rat auditory pathway [74]. Recently, AIM-MRI was transferred to transgenic mice to characterize sound-evoked and tone-specific activity patterns in *fibroblast growth factor 17* mutants [75].

Given the specific kinetics of Mn^{2+} turnover in the CNS, which implies accumulation within minutes to hours and retention for several days, the pattern of activation will be retained for a long time. Therefore, for all AIM-MRI experiments, the sensoric stimulation can be applied to awake animals outside the MR scanner where they behave in their normal environment. On the other hand, AIM-MRI is insensitive to the monitoring of rapid changes in neuronal activity, including deactivation patterns. However, once the animal is in the scanner, brain electrical activity is strongly dependent on the anesthetic level, which might affect the rate of further Mn^{2+} uptake and, therefore, the relative intensity of signal enhancement. Further experiments are necessary to determine the exact influence of scan duration and anesthetic depth on quantitative image acquisition in AIM-MRI.

The relationship between sensory stimulation and signal enhancement by AIM-MRI might not always be as straightforward as for the acoustic system. Previously, the accumulation of Mn^{2+} along the visual projection in light- or dark-adapted rodents has been investigated [47, 61]. In the retina, AIM-MRI reveals a shift in the layer-specific ion demand that is associated with light and dark visual processing by photoreceptor cells as well as interneurons and/or RGCs. More specifically, in rats that received an intraperitoneal injection of $MnCl_2$, dark current-dependent Mn^{2+} uptake into photoreceptor cells becomes substantially diminished under light stimulation, while concomitant uptake within the inner retinal layers modestly increases [47]. Thus, when measured on a clinical 3T scanner following intravitreal application of Mn^{2+}, the overall retinal signal intensity is more enhanced after dark adaptation, but not after light stimulation. To explore the consequences of illumination conditions for Mn^{2+} accumulation along the retino-tectal projection, Fischer and colleagues compared the signal enhancement in the LGN and SC. Surprisingly, they did not observe any differences in Mn^{2+}-dependent contrast enhancement in mice of both cohorts [61]. This might be explained by the presence of specialized, dark-responsive 'OFF-RGCs' and light-responsive 'ON-RGCs' in the retina and that their combined stimulation defines the net effect of electrical activity within the retino-tectal projection.

It is not yet fully understood which electrophysiological parameters, such as cellular depolarization, influence the transport and synaptic release of Mn^{2+}. As one of the first groups of researchers to utilize MEMRI to obtain genotype-phenotype correlations in transgenic mice, Bearer *et al.* (2007) analyzed the CBA mouse strain that is genetically blinded due to a lack of active photoreceptors [34]. Although there is no electrical activity along the optic nerve and the mice are visually impaired, they were still able to detect sufficient signal enhancement in the LGN and SC. Thus, axonal uptake and transport of Mn^{2+} can be uncoupled from electrical activity, but the latter might be necessary for its synaptic transmission [34]. Since the eye and the visual system offer a broad range of investigative tools that allows for functional and histological characterizations, this question might be resolved in the future.

Because AIM-MRI is sensitive to intracellular Ca^{2+} homeostasis, it should be responsive to pathological events that involve abnormal Ca^{2+} influx due to anoxic depolarization or excitotoxic release of glutamate. Several studies have tested AIM-MRI for its abilities to detect acute neuronal lesions or chronic neurodegeneration, such as after stroke, induced by neuroinflammation or during physiological aging [76-78]. They all show convincing results in support of its applicability as an early marker for aberrant Ca^{2+} influx. For example, when utilized in a rat model of permanent brain ischemia, AIM-MRI visualizes the ischemic core as early as 20 min after vascular occlusion [76]. Marked enhancements are observed in the lateral side of the caudate-putamen, and the lateral and ventral cortex including the piriform cortex (Figure 5). The hyperintensity area on Mn^{2+}-enhanced T_1-weighted images, which is caused by neuronal Ca^{2+} uptake related to the anoxic depolarization, is highly specific in differentiating the ischemic core from associated cortical areas compared to conventional MRI techniques such as DWI, T_2-weighted imaging, and apparent diffusion coefficient (ADC) [76]. Thus, AIM-MRI may be an additional technique to detect the penumbra in the ultra-early stage of brain ischemia.

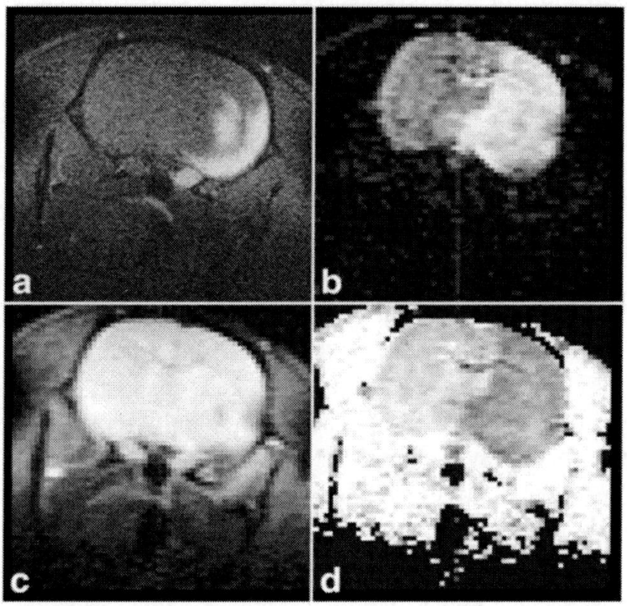

Figure 5. AIM-MRI application to detect neuronal activity in the neuropathological brain. Comparison of MEMRI, diffusion-weighted MRI (DWI), T_2-weighted imaging (T2W), and apparent diffusion coefficient (ADC) images of the same rat imaged on a 4.7T horizontal MR scanner 20 min after permanent cerebral occlusion. The high intensity area which localizes within the lateral side of the caudate-putamen and lateral cortex on MEMRI (a) is smaller than both DWI hyperintensity (b) and decreased ADC (d). A slight decreasing of the signal intensity is observed on the T2W image (c). [Adopted and reproduced from [76]. Reprinted with the permission of Wiley-Liss, Inc., a subsidiary of John Wiley & Sons, Inc.].

Limitations and Future Perspectives

While "the most important questions to be answered are whether acute and chronic toxicity are low enough to permit research and diagnosis on humans" [42] were raised as long as 30 years ago but have not yet been properly answered, MEMRI has found routine application in various experimental models of translational research. The evolution of this technique into a reliable neuroimaging method has been accompanied by improvements in MR scanner technology and the development of sophisticated pulse sequences enabling increased sensitivity and high spatial resolutions. A major drawback of the use of Mn^{2+} as a contrast agent in clinical diagnostics is its cellular toxicity. Besides circulatory failure and hepatic toxicity that are observed after acute overexposure to Mn^{2+}, severe neurotoxicity is caused by chronic contact or after topical applications at high dosages. The toxicity in the CNS is related to disturbances of Ca^{2+} homeostasis [79] and interference of Mn^{2+} with the mitochondrial respiratory chain, such as in clinically diagnosed Manganism [80]. Therefore, future goals for optimization of MEMRI will focus on the efficient delivery of Mn^{2+} to target structures by distinct topical loadings to circumvent systemic side effects. A promising approach is the application of Mn^{2+} solution as eye drops, e.g. for the diagnosis of retinal neuropathies. Initial results demonstrate the feasibility of topical loading to the cornea of 2 μl 1 M $MnCl_2$ to achieve retino-tectal signal enhancement as an alternative to intravitreal injections [81]. The method is sensitive in discriminating between intact and ischemic eyes, as indicated by a lack of signal enhancements in the optic nerve following retinal ischemia. Importantly, topical loading has been proven safe for repeated administrations and might be useful for monitoring retinal Mn^{2+} uptake and distribution as a measurement for retinal function in longitudinal studies [66]. Alternatively, systemic applications of Mn^{2+} derivatives are of great interest for diagnostic applications of MEMRI [82]. Thereby, the primary goal is to minimize the toxicity of Mn^{2+} by complexation and slow release into the target tissue. Various commercially available Mn^{2+}-based contrast agents, such as Teslascan® (GE Healthcare AS, Oslo, Norway) and SeeMore™ (Eagle Vision Pharmaceutical Corp, Exton, PA, USA), have been developed for clinical usage. Unfortunately, Teslascan® is currently withdrawn from the market in some countries due to unresolved side effects. However, new compounds, such as the intermediate-affinity chelate manganese *N*-(2-hydroxyethyl) iminodiacetic acid and silica-encapsulated $Mn_xFe_{1-x}O$ nanoparticles, are under development or are currently under investigation for their paramagnetic properties and biological tolerance [83-85].

Additionally, detailed knowledge of the biophysical properties of Mn^{2+} uptake, intracellular distribution, and metabolism is required to fully understand the principles behind Mn^{2+}-dependent signal enhancement for the different paradigms. For example, it is unclear how visual activity influences propagation of Mn^{2+} within the visual projection. In contrast to the acoustic system where Mn^{2+} accumulation within the inferior colliculi depends on acoustic stimulation [72], its propagation along the retino-tectal projection occurs independent of light or dark stimulation [61]. Moreover, given its applicability to the detection of aberrant Ca^{2+} influx under neuropathological conditions, a more detailed elucidation of the involved Ca^{2+} channels would certainly be of value for a more specific visualization and diagnosis of neuronal or axonal lesions not currently accessible by other contrast methods. Finally, it would be highly desirable to be able to detect Mn^{2+} tracing at the cellular or even subcellular level. This is achievable by X-ray fluorescence (XRF) microprobing of tissue samples. Thereby, a high-intensity focused X-ray beam causes manganese and other elements to fluoresce with a characteristic energy signature. In a recent study on Mn^{2+}-injected rats, *in vivo* MEMRI was combined with *post-mortem* XRF analysis of the Mn^{2+}-enhanced hippocampus. The maps of manganese distribution in CA3 and the dentate gyrus generated by the two techniques were found to overlay well, thus allowing usage of Mn^{2+} as a neuronal tract- or activity-specific tracer at the meso-scale level. It will be interesting to combine MEMRI and XRF data with histological methods to identify and characterize individual cells for their specific Mn^{2+} content [24]. Another approach for the histological detection of Mn^{2+} targets precipitation by autometallography [22, 61]. Superior to the resolution achieved by MEMRI, an increased concentration of manganese is found in deep cortical layers and within the piriform cortex in transgenic mice that lack the presynaptic active zone protein Bassoon [22]. However, prominent formation of the Mn^{2+} precipitate by sodium sulfide is missing in other areas of the brain that showed enhanced MEMRI signals in the *Bassoon knockout* mouse. Causative for the insensitivity of Mn-autometallography in these regions is the strong binding of Mn^{2+} to proteins that prevents the precipitation. This limitation might be overcome by increasing the dosage of Mn^{2+} to achieve saturation of protein binding.

Conclusion

In summary, the privileged entrance and distribution of systemically applied Mn^{2+} into the brain via the blood-brain barrier and ventricles, the ability for topical application by stereotaxic injection, the fast uptake into neurons through voltage-gated Ca^{2+} channels, the fast anterograde axonal transport and limited synaptic transmission, the long retention time in neuronal cells and tissues, together with the biological properties as a pivotal trace element and the paramagnetic properties make Mn^{2+} an ideal tracer for imaging brain anatomy, neuronal tracts, and neuronal activity. The kinetics of intracerebral threshold accumulation of Mn^{2+} allows for tracing and stimulation of animals several hours before the scan. Therefore, Mn^{2+} distribution occurs under normal physiological parameters of normally behaving animals. At the same time, the long retention time of Mn^{2+} disables the detection of fast changes in neuronal activity and contributes to the neurotoxicity that is, in particular, associated with higher dosages that are sometimes desired to gain additional MRI contrast. Upon resolution of these limitations, diagnostic MEMRI applications to monitor cerebral functions and neuropathological alterations in humans are clearly envisaged in the future.

Acknowledgments

Funding for this chapter was provided by the Leibniz Association, Germany and the Velux Foundation, Switzerland. I would like to thank Dr. K.-H. Herrmann (Institute of Diagnostic and Interventional Radiology I, Friedrich Schiller University of Jena Medical School) for inspiring scientific discussions and proofreading the chapter.

References

[1] Mori, S. and P.C. van Zijl, Fiber tracking: principles and strategies - a technical review. *NMR Biomed.*, 2002. 15(7-8): p. 468-80.

[2] Lee, S.K., et al., Diffusion-tensor MR imaging and fiber tractography: a new method of describing aberrant fiber connections in developmental CNS anomalies. *Radiographics,* 2005. 25(1): p. 53-65; discussion 66-8.

[3] Logothetis, N.K., The neural basis of the blood-oxygen-level-dependent functional magnetic resonance imaging signal. *Philos Trans. R. Soc. Lond B. Biol. Sci.,* 2002. 357(1424): p. 1003-37.

[4] Masamoto, K. and I. Kanno, Anesthesia and the quantitative evaluation of neurovascular coupling. *J. Cereb. Blood Flow Metab.*, 2012. 32(7): p. 1233-47.

[5] Silva, A.C. and N.A. Bock, Manganese-enhanced MRI: an exceptional tool in translational neuroimaging. *Schizophr. Bull.*, 2008. 34(4): p. 595-604.

[6] Kemmerer, A.R., C.A. Elvehjem, and E.B. Hart, Studies on the relation of manganese to the nutrition of the mouse. *J. Biol. Chem.*, 1931. 92: p. 623-630.

[7] Orent, E.R. and E.V. McCollum, Effects of deprivation of manganese in the rat. *J. Biol. Chem.*, 1931. 92(651-678).

[8] Roth, J.A. and M.D. Garrick, Iron interactions and other biological reactions mediating the physiological and toxic actions of manganese. *Biochem. Pharmacol.*, 2003. 66(1): p. 1-13.

[9] Chan, A.W., et al., Changes in brain regional manganese and magnesium levels during postnatal development: modulations by chronic manganese administration. *Metab. Brain Dis.,* 1992. 7(1): p. 21-33.

[10] Britton, A.A. and G.C. Cotzias, Dependence of manganese turnover on intake. *Am. J. Physiol.*, 1966. 211(1): p. 203-6.

[11] Thompson, T.N. and C.D. Klaassen, Presystemic elimination of manganese in rats. *Toxicol. Appl. Pharmacol.*, 1982. 64(2): p. 236-43.

[12] Crossgrove, J.S. and R.A. Yokel, Manganese distribution across the blood-brain barrier III. The divalent metal transporter-1 is not the major mechanism mediating brain manganese uptake. *Neurotoxicology*, 2004. 25(3): p. 451-60.

[13] Malecki, E.A., et al., Existing and emerging mechanisms for transport of iron and manganese to the brain. *J. Neurosci. Res.*, 1999. 56(2): p. 113-22.

[14] Narita, K., F. Kawasaki, and H. Kita, Mn and Mg influxes through Ca channels of motor nerve terminals are prevented by verapamil in frogs. *Brain Res.*, 1990. 510(2): p. 289-95.

[15] Drapeau, P. and D.A. Nachshen, Manganese fluxes and manganese-dependent neurotransmitter release in presynaptic nerve endings isolated from rat brain. *J. Physiol.*, 1984. 348: p. 493-510.

[16] Hankir, M.K., et al., The effects of glutamate receptor agonists and antagonists on mouse hypothalamic and hippocampal neuronal activity

shown through manganese enhanced MRI. *Neuroimage,* 2012. 59(2): p. 968-78.

[17] Dastur, D.K., D.K. Manghani, and K.V. Raghavendran, Distribution and fate of 54Mn in the monkey: studies of differnnt parts of the central nervous system and other organs. *J. Clin. Invest.*, 1971. 50(1): p. 9-20.

[18] Newland, M.C., et al., The clearance of manganese chloride in the primate. *Fundam. Appl. Toxicol.*, 1987. 9(2): p. 314-28.

[19] Qin, W.P., et al., [Variations of brain magnetic resonance imaging among manganese-exposed workers]. *Zhonghua Yu Fang Yi Xue Za Zhi*, 2009. 43(9): p. 793-7.

[20] Bock, N.A., F.F. Paiva, and A.C. Silva, Fractionated manganese-enhanced MRI. *NMR Biomed.*, 2008. 21(5): p. 473-8.

[21] Danscher, G. and J. Zimmer, An improved Timm sulphide silver method for light and electron microscopic localization of heavy metals in biological tissues. *Histochemistry*, 1978. 55(1): p. 27-40.

[22] Angenstein, F., et al., Manganese-enhanced MRI reveals structural and functional changes in the cortex of Bassoon mutant mice. *Cereb. Cortex*, 2007. 17(1): p. 28-36.

[23] Moldovan, N., et al., Altered transition metal homeostasis in mice following manganese injections for manganese-enhanced magnetic resonance imaging. *Biometals,* 2013. 26(1): p. 179-87.

[24] Daoust, A., E.L. Barbier, and S. Bohic, Manganese enhanced MRI in rat hippocampus: a correlative study with synchrotron X-ray microprobe. *Neuroimage*, 2013. 64: p. 10-8.

[25] Dastur, D.K., et al., Distribution and fate of Mn54 in the rat, with special reference to the C.N.S. *Q J. Exp. Physiol. Cogn. Med. Sci.*, 1969. 54(3): p. 322-31.

[26] Josephs, K.A., et al., Neurologic manifestations in welders with pallidal MRI T1 hyperintensity. *Neurology*, 2005. 64(12): p. 2033-9.

[27] Stredrick, D.L., et al., Manganese-induced cytotoxicity in dopamine-producing cells. *Neurotoxicology,* 2004. 25(4): p. 543-53.

[28] Cotzias, G.C., et al., Chronic manganese poisoning. Clearance of tissue manganese concentrations with persistance of the neurological picture. *Neurology*, 1968. 18(4): p. 376-82.

[29] Lewis, J., et al., Trigeminal uptake and clearance of inhaled manganese chloride in rats and mice. *Neurotoxicology*, 2005. 26(1): p. 113-23.

[30] Sidoryk-Wegrzynowicz, M. and M. Aschner, Role of astrocytes in manganese mediated neurotoxicity. *BMC Pharmacol. Toxicol.*, 2013. 14: p. 23.

[31] Canals, S., et al., Magnetic resonance imaging of cortical connectivity in vivo. *Neuroimage,* 2008. 40(2): p. 458-72.

[32] Tjalve, H., et al., Uptake of manganese and cadmium from the nasal mucosa into the central nervous system via olfactory pathways in rats. *Pharmacol. Toxicol.,* 1996. 79(6): p. 347-56.

[33] Sloot, W.N. and J.B. Gramsbergen, Axonal transport of manganese and its relevance to selective neurotoxicity in the rat basal ganglia. *Brain Res.*, 1994. 657(1-2): p. 124-32.

[34] Bearer, E.L., et al., Role of neuronal activity and kinesin on tract tracing by manganese-enhanced MRI (MEMRI). *Neuroimage,* 2007. 37 Suppl 1: p. S37-46.

[35] Takeda, A., Manganese action in brain function. *Brain Res. Brain Res. Rev.*, 2003. 41(1): p. 79-87.

[36] Lauffer, R.B., Targeted relaxation enhancement agents for MRI. *Magn. Reson. Med.,* 1991. 22(2): p. 339-42; discussion 343-6.

[37] Silva, A.C., et al., Manganese-enhanced magnetic resonance imaging (MEMRI): methodological and practical considerations. *NMR Biomed.*, 2004. 17(8): p. 532-43.

[38] Nordhoy, W., et al., Manganese ions as intracellular contrast agents: proton relaxation and calcium interactions in rat myocardium. *NMR Biomed.*, 2003. 16(2): p. 82-95.

[39] Lee, J.H., et al., Manganese-enhanced magnetic resonance imaging of mouse brain after systemic administration of $MnCl_2$: dose-dependent and temporal evolution of T1 contrast. *Magn. Reson. Med.*, 2005. 53(3): p. 640-8.

[40] Haenold, R., et al., Magnetic resonance imaging of the mouse visual pathway for in vivo studies of degeneration and regeneration in the CNS. *Neuroimage*, 2012. 59(1): p. 363-76.

[41] Lauterbur, P., Image formation by induced local interactions: examples employing nuclear magnetic resonance. *Nature*, 1973. 242: p. 2.

[42] Mendonca-Dias, M.H., E. Gaggelli, and P.C. Lauterbur, Paramagnetic contrast agents in nuclear magnetic resonance medical imaging. *Semin. Nucl. Med.,* 1983. 13(4): p. 364-76.

[43] Newland, M.C., et al., Visualizing manganese in the primate basal ganglia with magnetic resonance imaging. *Exp. Neurol.*, 1989. 106(3): p. 251-8.

[44] Lin, Y.J. and A.P. Koretsky, Manganese ion enhances T1-weighted MRI during brain activation: an approach to direct imaging of brain function. *Magn. Reson. Med.* 1997. 38(3): p. 378-88.

[45] Pautler, R.G., A.C. Silva, and A.P. Koretsky, In vivo neuronal tract tracing using manganese-enhanced magnetic resonance imaging. *Magn. Reson. Med.*, 1998. 40(5): p. 740-8.
[46] Koretsky, A.P. and A.C. Silva, Manganese-enhanced magnetic resonance imaging (MEMRI). *NMR Biomed.*, 2004. 17(8): p. 527-31.
[47] Berkowitz, B.A., et al., Noninvasive and simultaneous imaging of layer-specific retinal functional adaptation by manganese-enhanced MRI. *Invest. Ophthalmol. Vis. Sci.*, 2006. 47(6): p. 2668-74.
[48] Aoki, I., et al., In vivo detection of neuroarchitecture in the rodent brain using manganese-enhanced MRI. *Neuroimage*, 2004. 22(3): p. 1046-59.
[49] London, R.E., et al., Magnetic resonance imaging studies of the brains of anesthetized rats treated with manganese chloride. *Brain Res. Bull.*, 1989. 23(3): p. 229-35.
[50] Watanabe, T., et al., In vivo 3D MRI staining of mouse brain after subcutaneous application of MnCl2. *Magn. Reson. Med.*, 2002. 48(5): p. 852-9.
[51] Bock, N.A., et al., Cerebrospinal fluid to brain transport of manganese in a non-human primate revealed by MRI. *Brain Res.*, 2008. 1198: p. 160-70.
[52] Szulc, K.U., et al., MRI analysis of cerebellar and vestibular developmental phenotypes in Gbx2 conditional knockout mice. *Magn. Reson. Med.,* 2013.
[53] Watanabe, T., J. Frahm, and T. Michaelis, Myelin mapping in the living mouse brain using manganese-enhanced magnetization transfer MRI. *Neuroimage*, 2010. 49(2): p. 1200-4.
[54] Watanabe, T., J. Frahm, and T. Michaelis, Myelin mapping in the central nervous system of living mice using contrast-enhanced magnetization transfer MRI. *Neuroimage*, 2012. 63(2): p. 812-7.
[55] Watanabe, T., J. Frahm, and T. Michaelis, Functional mapping of neural pathways in rodent brain in vivo using manganese-enhanced three-dimensional magnetic resonance imaging. *NMR Biomed.*, 2004. 17(8): p. 554-68.
[56] Tjalve, H., C. Mejare, and K. Borg-Neczak, Uptake and transport of manganese in primary and secondary olfactory neurones in pike. *Pharmacol. Toxicol.*, 1995. 77(1): p. 23-31.
[57] Takeda, A., et al., Manganese transport in the neural circuit of rat CNS. *Brain Res. Bull.*, 1998. 45(2): p. 149-52.
[58] Henriksson, J., J. Tallkvist, and H. Tjalve, Transport of manganese via the olfactory pathway in rats: dosage dependency of the uptake and

subcellular distribution of the metal in the olfactory epithelium and the brain. *Toxicol. Appl. Pharmacol.*, 1999. 156(2): p. 119-28.
[59] Watanabe, T., T. Michaelis, and J. Frahm, Mapping of retinal projections in the living rat using high-resolution 3D gradient-echo MRI with Mn2+-induced contrast. *Magn. Reson. Med.*, 2001. 46(3): p. 424-9.
[60] Thuen, M., et al., Manganese-enhanced MRI of the optic visual pathway and optic nerve injury in adult rats. *J. Magn. Reson. Imaging*, 2005. 22(4): p. 492-500.
[61] Fischer, S., et al., In vivo Imaging of Optic Nerve Fiber Integrity by Contrast-enhanced MRI in Mice. *J. Vis. Exp.*, 2013.
[62] Chan, K.C. and E.X. Wu, In vivo manganese-enhanced MRI for visuotopic brain mapping. *Conf Proc IEEE Eng. Med. Biol. Soc.*, 2012. 2012: p. 2279-82.
[63] Chan, K.C., et al., In vivo retinotopic mapping of superior colliculus using manganese-enhanced magnetic resonance imaging. *Neuroimage,* 2011. 54(1): p. 389-95.
[64] Thuen, M., et al., Combination of Mn(2+)-enhanced and diffusion tensor MR imaging gives complementary information about injury and regeneration in the adult rat optic nerve. *J. Magn. Reson. Imaging*, 2009. 29(1): p. 39-51.
[65] Sandvig, I., et al., In vivo MRI of olfactory ensheathing cell grafts and regenerating axons in transplant mediated repair of the adult rat optic nerve. *NMR Biomed.*, 2012. 25(4): p. 620-31.
[66] Sun, S.W., T. Thiel, and H.F. Liang, Impact of repeated topical-loaded manganese-enhanced MRI on the mouse visual system. *Invest. Ophthalmol. Vis. Sci.*, 2012. 53(8): p. 4699-709.
[67] Cross, D.J., et al., Age-related decrease in axonal transport measured by MR imaging in vivo. *Neuroimage,* 2008. 39(3): p. 915-26.
[68] Smith, K.D., et al., In vivo axonal transport rates decrease in a mouse model of Alzheimer's disease. *Neuroimage*, 2007. 35(4): p. 1401-8.
[69] Kim, J., et al., Quantitative in vivo measurement of early axonal transport deficits in a triple transgenic mouse model of Alzheimer's disease using manganese-enhanced MRI. *Neuroimage*, 2011. 56(3): p. 1286-92.
[70] Bertrand, A., et al., Non-invasive, in vivo monitoring of neuronal transport impairment in a mouse model of tauopathy using MEMRI. *Neuroimage,* 2013. 64: p. 693-702.

[71] Duong, T.Q., et al., Functional MRI of calcium-dependent synaptic activity: cross correlation with CBF and BOLD measurements. *Magn. Reson. Med.*, 2000. 43(3): p. 383-92.
[72] Yu, X., et al., In vivo auditory brain mapping in mice with Mn-enhanced MRI. *Nat. Neurosci.*, 2005. 8(7): p. 961-8.
[73] Watanabe, T., J. Frahm, and T. Michaelis, Manganese-enhanced MRI of the mouse auditory pathway. *Magn. Reson. Med.*, 2008. 60(1): p. 210-2.
[74] Jin, S.U., et al., Intratympanic manganese administration revealed sound intensity and frequency dependent functional activity in rat auditory pathway. *Magn. Reson. Imaging*, 2013.
[75] Yu, X., et al., Morphological and functional midbrain phenotypes in Fibroblast Growth Factor 17 mutant mice detected by Mn-enhanced MRI. *Neuroimage,* 2011. 56(3): p. 1251-8.
[76] Aoki, I., et al., Detection of the anoxic depolarization of focal ischemia using manganese-enhanced MRI. *Magn. Reson. Med.*, 2003. 50(1): p. 7-12.
[77] Boretius, S., et al., MRI of optic neuritis in a rat model. *Neuroimage,* 2008. 41(2): p. 323-34.
[78] Bissig, D., D. Goebel, and B.A. Berkowitz, Diminished vision in healthy aging is associated with increased retinal L-type voltage gated calcium channel ion influx. *PLoS One*, 2013. 8(2): p. e56340.
[79] Aschner, M. and J.L. Aschner, Manganese transport across the blood-brain barrier: relationship to iron homeostasis. *Brain Res. Bull.*, 1990. 24(6): p. 857-60.
[80] Santamaria, A.B., Manganese exposure, essentiality & toxicity. *Indian J. Med. Res.*, 2008. 128(4): p. 484-500.
[81] Sun, S.W., et al., Noninvasive topical loading for manganese-enhanced MRI of the mouse visual system. *Invest. Ophthalmol. Vis. Sci.*, 2011. 52(6): p. 3914-20.
[82] Tofts, P.S., et al., Toward clinical application of manganese-enhanced MRI of retinal function. *Brain Res. Bull.*, 2010. 81(2-3): p. 333-8.
[83] Bertin, A., et al., Development of a dendritic manganese-enhanced magnetic resonance imaging (MEMRI) contrast agent: synthesis, toxicity (in vitro) and relaxivity (in vitro, in vivo) studies. *Bioconjug. Chem.,* 2009. 20(4): p. 760-7.
[84] Seo, Y., et al., Mn-citrate and Mn-HIDA: intermediate-affinity chelates for manganese-enhanced MRI. *Contrast Media Mol. Imaging*, 2013. 8(2): p. 140-6.

[85] Chen, W., et al., Manganese-enhanced MRI of rat brain based on slow cerebral delivery of manganese(II) with silica-encapsulated Mnx Fe1-x O nanoparticles. *NMR Biomed.*, 2013. 26(9): p. 1176-85.

Index

#

A

B

C

D

E

F

G

H

I

J

K

L

M

N

O

P

Q

R

S

T

U

V

W